UNDE
CANDIDA

UNDERSTANDING CANDIDA:
treatment and recipes

Peter de Ruyter

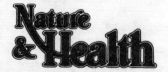

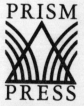

THIS BOOK IS NOT INTENDED FOR SELF-DIAGNOSIS OR TREATMENT. IT IS WRITTEN AS A GUIDE ONLY. PLEASE CONSULT YOUR PRACTITIONER BEFORE TAKING ANY MEDICINES MENTIONED HERE, OR BEFORE CONSIDERING THERAPY.

First published in Australasia in 1989 by
Nature & Health Books
This edition co-published in Great Britain by
Prism Press, 2 South Street, Bridport,
Dorset DT6 3NQ, England
and distributed in the United States of America by
the Avery Publishing Group Inc.,
350 Thorens Avenue, Garden City Park, New York, 11040

ISBN 1 85327 035 0 (Prism Press) ISBN 0 949099 14 7 (Nature & Health Books)

Copyright © 1989 Peter de Ruyter

All rights reserved, no part of this publication may be reproduced, stored in a retrieval system, transmitted in any form or by any means, electronic, mechanical, photocopying, recording or otherwise, without the prior permission in writing of the publisher.

Printed by The Guernsey Press, Guernsey, Channel Islands.

CONTENTS

Acknowledgements	
Preface	
Background information to help understand the basis to the Candida diet and therapy	5
A brief overview of Candida	7
But is it simply Candida?	11
How Candida can be specifically diagnosed	17
Naturopathic views of why disease occurs	23
How Candida *can* be beaten!	27
Extra dimensions to Candida therapy	33
When I am well again . . .	41
Detailed explanations of the Candida diet	45
Responsibility and healing: inseparable companions	47
The anti-Candida diet: a basis to your therapy	49
The anti-Candida diet: what *can* I eat?	55
The anti-Candida diet: what *can't* I eat?	63
Recipes and further hints	67
Information on the 14-day rotation diet	69
Shopping list for Week I	73
Menu for Week I: Breakfast, Lunch, Dinner	77
Shopping list for Week II	97
Menu for Week II: Breakfast, Lunch, Dinner	99
Salads, Snack Foods, Sauces and more!	115
EPILOGUE	131
APPENDIX	133
BIBLIOGRAPHY	139

This book is dedicated to Harry.

ACKNOWLEDGEMENTS

A special thanks must go firstly to my many clients who, through their persistent questioning, made me realise the need for a book such as this. Then to Chanelle McKellar for stimulating me into finally doing something about it. To Harry Binder for his help in the cooking section, constantly coming up with useful hints and advice, and for his commitment in supporting me in so many ways whilst writing this book. To Clive Chappell, not only for his help in the cooking section, but especially for his tremendous clarity in doing the proofreading. To Chris Harris for his much appreciated cooking hints, and to Pippa Preston for her numerous recipes.

PREFACE

In this book I won't go into fine detail of exactly what Candidiasis is all about. Too many other marvellous books exist which go into great depth on this topic, and it is highly recommended that, at least, *The Yeast Connection* by W. Crook MD be read if you are a lay person, and *The Missing Diagnosis* by Orion Truss MD, if more scientifically inclined. In fact, if that is your bent, then I would suggest reading Appendix I and II of *The Missing Diagnosis*, before reading the rest of the book. This advice would be especially applicable if at all sceptical about the whole issue of Candidiasis as a basis of ill-health in people, young or old, male or female.

These two texts are the original classics on the subject, but as can be seen from the bibliography, many more books have been written on this extraordinarily important topic over the last three to five years. Another most convincing scientific piece of work to read for the sceptical is included in the book by Brostoff and Challacombe, *Food Allergy and Intolerance*, chapter 49. Much research exists in published form if one chooses to look for it, and it becomes impossible to discount the Candida issue.

This book therefore is written, not necessarily to prove the reality of Candidiasis, but rather to answer a need voiced so frequently by many of my clients. Although they were given the diet sheet and this was thoroughly explained during the initial diagnosis and consultation, many nevertheless were so overcome by the deluge of new information — much of it shaking their existing lifestyles right to the core — that they felt helpless and lost once they went home and had, in many cases, to look at totally rethinking and reorganising that everyday lifestyle.

One of the major problems was, of course, the utterly confusing amount of conflict, contradiction and controversy that unfortunately is associated with the subject of Candida. Not just about whether it exists, but also about treatment. Every practitioner seems to have their own pet way of dealing with Candida, each claiming to have *the* answer which cures.

Yet, when you look at all the books available, especially cookbooks, it doesn't take long to realise that serious contradictions exist. One recipe or practitioner will allow juice for example; the other will definitely say no! So, for you, the person with Candida as a health issue, who is right? Everyone you read or speak to seems to have 'evidence', research data, double-blind, placebo-controlled trials to prove that *their* information is correct.

That was the major reason why, for years, I did not want anything to do with the subject of Candida. It was too much of a hot 'therapeutic' potato. But then circumstances — the severe illness of a friend who was being treated for Candida

— forced me to re-evaluate the whole issue. Witnessing the controversy surrounding the treatment of this friend for Candida, and seeing the obvious harm his Candida program was doing to him, made me want to look deeper. I had to admit that he did have Candida, and that yes, it *does* exist as a real disease, rather than as a figment of some fevered imagination.

About that time I had gone overseas to the US and Holland, and while there I decided to gather as much information as I could. When I returned, I combined it with all the data I had already accumulated here. I next spent weeks going through this mountain of literature, trying to find the common thread. And out of this laborious melting pot came my own anti-Candida program of diet and treatment.

The next hurdle was to see if this approach would work, and after two years and hundreds of cases of Candida, I feel secure in saying that my views and techniques *do* work. However, let it be clearly understood that I am not saying that this is the ultimate truth on how to treat Candida. There are many ways of skinning a cat, and this is only my way, but hopefully a way that excludes a lot of fanaticism and extremes that I've encountered in so many other approaches.

I make a point of trying to give a rational explanation for why I suggest the therapeutic approaches I do. Knowledge gives people more power to stick to regimes that are otherwise quite contrary to what they have followed in the past. And finally, it is of the utmost importance that people learn to listen and attend to what *their* bodies are telling them.

In other words, it's all very well to have a wonderful diet and therapeutic regime worked out but one cannot say, "Ah, here is *the* Candida treatment which now can be universally applied." It would be far more accurate to say, "Here is *one* Candida approach that can be adapted to the individual's needs."

This is a point that is all too frequently missed in any therapy. There simply cannot be a 'standard' treatment. Show me a 'standard' human being, and then I'll be only too happy to prescribe such a treatment! Herein of course lies the confusion surrounding Candida therapy: there needs to be as many approaches to treatment as there are individual, non-standard people.

The problem therefore is the inflexibility of therapists, as much as the rest of society, to appreciate this fact. They need to allow their approach to treatment to be just a basis from which adaptations can then be made, as circumstances dictate.

So if anyone wants to query my approach, that is good. But let the final judgement rest upon the results obtained, by following the program for a reasonable period of time (for at least 4-6 months initially). If it works, great! If not satisfied, that is okay too and something that does suit *your* individual needs must be found elsewhere.

PREFACE

I feel my own views and protocols will continue to change or evolve as new experience or data comes to hand. And this is obviously as it should be, rather than dogmatically remaining caught in the rut of 'how it was all done'.

Enough philosophy then, and on to the more practical aspects of this book. The best way of dealing with old, destructive habits is to learn to replace them with new, constructive ones. A major problem encountered by my clients was that they were stuck in old patterns which were usually the reason why they developed Candida in the first place. To be told suddenly that they need to drop this and change that, leaves a nasty vacuum in life.

"What is there left to eat?", "None of my recipes are applicable anymore!", "I don't know what to cook!" These and many more are the desperate, often angry comments that I hear shortly after most clients start their program. The fact that many so-called 'yeast-free' cookbooks often clash with my dietary directions doesn't help either.

The fundamental idea here is to provide a two-week rotational, very simple and basic dietary roster that gives people dealing with Candida an initial step-by-step guide to what *can* still be eaten.

This book or this program is not to be seen as the definitive work on yeast-free cooking. Many more recipes exist or could be modified or invented that would very adequately cater for all types of tastes. Most people suffering from Candida are busy, working people who have little time (or energy!) to prepare difficult or elaborate meals.

One major symptom of Candida is 'fuzzy-headedness', the inability to think or plan. So to devise a yeast-free, sugar-free meal for tonight, or for lunch or breakfast, is already too much, let alone planning for all meals over a one-week period.

Hence this basic, two-week program. Firstly, the aim is to provide good, properly balanced nutrition that involves all the food groups: proteins, complex carbohydrate, vegetables, fats and oils and eventually fruit. Since Candida is not treated overnight, it means that people need to remain on this type of diet for many months.

It therefore becomes imperative that any diet used is one that is nutritionally sound and balanced, and will not result in deficiencies or problems over time, as so many Candida diets do. Certain foods, especially for breakfast, are rotated as much as possible to avoid the real possibility of creating allergies or food-sensitivity reactions.

Shopping lists are provided for the program, one week in advance, to cater for all your meals for each week. Once the two weeks have been completed, either start Week I again, or begin to experiment a little yourself within the boundaries set out later in this book.

UNDERSTANDING CANDIDA

For the initial period of adjustment to these changes in your life (post-Candida diagnosis!), you now have a step-by-step, simple and nutritious program to follow.

I trust this book fulfils your needs and hope that the issue of Candida in your life can be seen as an adventure. Like the glass which has water in it to the half-way mark, this can be seen as half empty *or* as half full. The reality remains exactly the same, but your perception of it can greatly affect how you experience that reality. Truly, that choice can only be made by you.

See it, therefore, as a wonderful — albeit confronting — opportunity to experience new, constructive dimensions in your life.

Good luck!

Bondi
July 1988

SECTION I

Background information to help understand the basis to the Candida diet and therapy

1 A BRIEF OVERVIEW OF CANDIDA

Two areas that seem to need an enormous amount of explaining when people first hear about Candida are: 'What is it?' and 'Why is my doctor so sceptical about it?' If the first question is adequately answered, then the reason for the second becomes more predictable: we realise that many doctors, laypeople and even natural therapists are under an unfortunate misapprehension.

The crucial point to understand is that Candida exists in at least two different forms. Everyone, young and old, male and female has within their gut a type of yeast called *Candida albicans*. It is precisely the same organism that can cause vaginal thrush, or oral thrush which is often seen in babies. Hence, from this point of view, doctors or sceptics are totally correct when, to a client who comes to them with the comments, "My natural therapist says I have Candida", they answer with scorn, "Of course you have Candida . . . and so have I!!"

With such a flippant remark they hope to make that the end of the matter. They regard such a diagnosis as just quackery and as something that needs to be discounted as quickly and thoroughly as possible. The fact is that it isn't quite so simple. Yes, everyone *does* have Candida in their gut, but what *form* is it in? This organism is able to exist in at least two distinct forms: as a yeast and as a disease-causing fungus.

This difference may seem too insignificant to be concerned about, and yet this is what the whole Candida-as-a-disease issue hinges on. The ironic thing is that all the research that has been done on Candida — and there is a large amount of it! — has been done by very learned scientists and doctors with excellent qualifications. It has been done in their laboratories and then written up in their prestigious scientific or medical journals. The sad thing is that many doctors don't read their own journals . . . but many natural therapists do! And they have applied what they have read into practise, with excellent results.

No longer can it be denied that Candida in the pathogenic (disease-causing) form can be the basis to an extraordinary amount of suffering, creating symptoms not only on physical levels, but on mental and emotional ones too.

So, let's briefly look at how and why this is so. Normally, Candida in the yeast form lives very happily in our gut, along with all the other bacteria that usually live there. Everything is in an 'ecological balance'. However, there are many reasons why this delicate balance can be upset, and, when this happens, the yeast changes into a fungus which can be very aggressive and is able to spread rapidly, not only within the bowels themselves, but even beyond the bowel wall.

Our Western society is an ideal breeding ground for creating such imbalances in our gut ecology. Indeed, if we had actively set out to develop a Candida problem in a population, it couldn't have been carried out in more ideal circumstances than the ones we find ourselves in today.

One of the most important factors in setting the scene for a Candida transformation and take over, is the indiscriminate abuse of anti-biotics. They certainly have their value in life-threatening illnesses but, as with all 'magic bullets', they exact a price from our bodies. Antibiotics don't necessarily kill only the specific infection for which they were prescribed, they can also have a profound effect on the friendly bacteria in our gut.

Anti-biotics do *not* affect Candida, as it is a yeast, not a bacterium. The Candida then finds itself in the position of a cleaned-out gut, where there are no longer enough — if any — bacteria left to keep it in check. Within days, the Candida can change from its yeast form into the fungal, disease-causing form which then rapidly spreads throughout the gut and beyond.

It is in this form that the Candida can produce a complex network of highly potent toxins or poisons (over 70 of these have been isolated and researched in laboratories). These are slowly released in its day-to-day growth and it is these poisons that can so profoundly affect every organ and gland in our entire body. This is why a Candida infestation can result in such a variety of symptoms, affecting not only the physical body, but the emotional and mental parts of us, too.

Some of these toxins have a direct immunosuppressive action: the fungus maintains its 'take-over' situation in the body, by paralysing the defences produced by the immune system, that would otherwise bring the situation back under control. This is obviously significant to the safety and health of the body on other levels too, because a paralysed or disabled immune system means that the body then becomes far more susceptible to all types of other infections, auto-immune problems, cancers and more.

So antibiotics are probably the worst offenders in setting up a Candida problem. Just think for a moment about how often antibiotics have been prescribed in your life, or to someone close to you. All too frequently they are prescribed for the flu (which is due to a virus and therefore unaffected by antibiotics!).

Fungi — like Candida — and viruses, cannot be killed by normal antibiotics. There are not many people in our society today who haven't had at least one course of antibiotics in their life. And, for some people who have a sensitive gut-balance between the bacteria and yeast, it need take only *one* course to throw them into an unbalanced ecology, that is, full-blown, disease-causing Candida.

A BRIEF OVERVIEW OF CANDIDA

Think about all the people who have had antibiotics — often for years — for a chronic acne problem. Even for those of you who think you've never had an antibiotic, think again, because there are traces of antibiotics in most meats, poultry and eggs, due to the foods fed to animals. Over time, in some sensitive people, this alone can cause Candida overgrowth.

Then there are factors such as cortisone, high sugar diets, stress, insufficient secretion of stomach acids, the Pill, hormonal replacement in women who have had total hysterectomies or are going through menopause, and even those who have had many pregnancies. All these factors have the ability to affect Candida overgrowth in our gut: there would be very few people who would not have been exposed to at least one of these influences; most of us are exposed to several, and over a long period of time! In this category, diets high in sugar would be the worst.

Is it therefore *really* so surprising to discover that we have epidemic proportions of Candida in our Western, high-tech society? So many people feel that Candida is the 'in' disease to have, that it's the 'flavour of the month'. On one level this may seem to be so. However, by looking a little deeper at the situation it becomes obvious that despite the number of 'authorities' who may wish to remain blind to the facts and continue to insist that it is all a fad, the stark truth is that Candida is very much a serious problem in our society. This problem is also likely to become worse before it gets better, simply because the factors creating Candida overgrowth are not lessening. They are increasing, although in some segments of our society there is a growing awareness of the root of this condition, and therefore a willingness to change.

AIDS seems to be the big issue at present, and with reason. But I would suggest that Candida will be seen as possibly an even greater creator of suffering, in times ahead, simply because of the far greater numbers that are *already* affected by it but, tragically, have not yet been diagnosed. They continue to go from doctor to doctor to specialist, then often to natural therapists, and yet nothing can be found. The ultimate conclusion? 'As all the tests are normal, there can be nothing wrong with you, so it's all in your head. You need a psychiatrist!'

With all due respect to psychiatrists, all of us have some skeletons in our closet, which no doubt will be prised out and held up as the reason for all our symptoms, especially for the unlucky sufferers of Candida who tend to get a lot of mental or emotional symptoms. But working on this level will never get to the root cause of the Candida-based symptoms.

Yet, Candida *is* treatable!

2 BUT IS IT SIMPLY CANDIDA?

The problem with Candida is that the symptoms found in this condition can be mimicked to a great extent by various other ill-health states, such as hypoglycaemia, allergies, hypothyroidism or post-viral syndrome. At the bottom of all of these usually lies a malfunctioning or underfunctioning immune system.

And you thought Candida alone was complicated? My experience has time after time proven that, in ill-health, nothing is ever simple, black or white. Often, there are several factors interacting to give the overall disease picture of symptoms. The aim is to untangle these different components and treat them appropriately. To just treat a condition, any condition, symptomatically, is asking for a long and difficult recovery.

One or two symptoms may go, but the most important factor will have been overlooked: 'What was the root cause of those symptoms in the first place?' Treat the condition from this perspective, and the whole situation will shift. Miss it, and you'll be playing 'musical symptoms' because no sooner will one disappear, than another will pop up somewhere else, simply because the *source* of the symptoms hasn't been looked at.

Most of you will know what a pest the noxious weed privet can be. This is a plant that you can continue to prune or even chop back. But unless you actually dig out the roots, it will continue to come up again. This is the whole point of symptomatic treatment (band-aid jobs) versus holistic treatment (treating the cause, not *only* the symptoms).

Hence, for therapists it is already bad enough trying to diagnose all the possible levels to a particular client's range of presenting symptoms. For the layperson to try to do so can be folly. Some progress certainly can be made, but until the complete — or as complete as possible — picture can be elicited, treatment results are often very haphazard. For this, a good holistically inclined therapist is essential. It is not so much that they then cure you, but rather that they can reflect back at you a far more accurate picture of where you, with your particular health problem, are stuck. And then you, armed with this deeper and broader view, with also deeper and broader treatment regimes, can go ahead to *cure yourself*. We as therapists never cure. Only you do that, although we certainly act as 'mirrors' to allow you to see more clearly where you may be stuck. We act as guides to the best 'treatment road' for you to follow. This is an important twist of emphasis that is vital to understand if true healing is to be achieved. This point will be expanded upon later.

So, it is most important to realise that, when you read about Candida in a book or article or hear someone speak about it, it can be very seductive and easy to assume that you too have Candida. If your symptoms fit those commonly ascribed to Candida, then it is likely that you have Candida — if not as the totality of your situation, then at least as part of your problem. But there may be more to it than that.

Let's look closer at the complicating factors. Hypoglycaemia is often seen to be associated with Candida simply because the toxins released by the Candida fungus can create wild fluctuations in your blood sugars. Your natural therapist who does iridology will be able to differentiate between 'pure' hypoglycaemia and Candida, or, alternatively, decide whether your 'hypoglycaemic' symptoms are more due to the Candida in the first place. This can be seen from certain signs in the iris corresponding to the liver, pancreas, adrenal, thyroid and stomach zones.

To an extent, it is more of a philosophical nicety here, as the Candida diet very adequately controls hypoglycaemic symptoms, too. Where it does become important to distinguish between these two factors as the possible source to your symptoms is in herbal treatment. There are very potent and healing herbs that can be used in treating a true hypoglycaemic condition, such as Dandelion, Licorice, Fennel, Juniper, Wild Yam, Meadowsweet or Blue Flag. Again, there is never a 'standard' remedy for any condition, so it is important to have the guidance of a holistic therapist, preferably a herbalist, to choose the most appropriate remedy for your individual situation.

Since the Candida fungus is able to penetrate the bowel walls, it creates 'leaks' as it were, allowing partially digested food particles to seep through, acting then as foreign intruders in your inner body. This automatically sets off alarm bells and the body's immune defences rush to the scene. In doing so, an allergic or food sensitivity reaction can be experienced within you.

Because we eat at least three times a day, and because such reactions can happen frequently in someone with Candida, the immune system becomes more and more exhausted with time. This leaves the Candida unchallenged in your body and allows it to spread further and more aggressively.

It is important to minimise allergic reactions as much as possible. Some therapists do so by putting people with multiple allergies on the most extraordinarily restrictive diets which, after a while, result in malnourishment and further weakening of your body. This is yet another example of symptomatic treatment. By all means take out the most obvious and severely reacting foods, but it is of vital importance to maintain as full a balanced and nourishing a diet as possible.

Rotation of foods (as in the diet discussed later) plus treating the body on deeper levels (also discussed later) will overcome these problems in time.

The next factor to look at is hypothyroidism. This is a subject that could take an

BUT IS IT SIMPLY CANDIDA?

entire book to discuss. In fact such a book exists in Broda Barnes's *Hypothyroidism — The Unsuspected Illness*. Barnes describes a level of thyroid *under*function that is rarely picked up. The blood tests for thyroid function only really pick up *mal*function, and will not show up the typical underfunctioning thyroid that, nevertheless, can be the basis of a vast range of symptoms. It is also directly implicated in the Candida situation in that an underfunctioning thyroid automatically means an underfunctioning immune system. This in turn makes it easier for the Candida to spread in the body, wreaking havoc.

There is however a very, very simple test that anyone can do to see if the thyroid is implicated in your Candida problem: take a thermometer and shake it down thoroughly the night before you decide to do the test. Leave it close to your bedside where you can reach it easily the next morning with a minimum of movement. The vital point here is to take your temperature *underarm*, first thing upon awakening in the morning. Lie as still as a corpse for ten minutes, by the clock. Only then may you get up and do whatever you need to do. This process should preferably be repeated for three consecutive mornings to give a consistent and average temperature reading.

For menstruating women, it should only be done on the second, third and fourth morning after they have commenced their period. If you have had a partial hysterectomy and feel your ovaries are still active, then try and "feel" when you might normally have had your period, taking the temperature then. If you are unable to "feel" this event, then you will need to take your temperature every morning for a full month.

The whole aim of this procedure is to find what the lowest temperature is your body produces, not only within a 24 hour cycle, but also within a monthly cycle. This is termed your "basal metabolic temperature" and this is often called the "B.M.T. Test".

If the temperature is less than 36.5 degrees Celcius, then you have a measure of hypothyroidism, in the sense that your thyroid is UNDERfunctioning, not MALfunctioning. This in turn is of great importance in the overall treatment, whether you have Candida or any other problem, as adequate thyroid function is also most important in regulating normal blood sugar levels ie. hypoglycaemia. Thyroid malfunction can be another important basis to allergy problems. Also, by affecting immune function, it allows Candida to proliferate. These are only some of the vital roles that thyroid function is implicated in, but it is enough to show how any symptoms a person is presenting with needs to be looked at very closely, rather than just assuming that the problem is ONLY Candida, or ONLY hypoglycaemia, etc.

Indeed, treating ONLY on that level will result in some improvements, but for really deep healing changes to occur, all these possibilities at least need to be looked at. In this way, these factors can either be dismissed as not being implicated in this particular client's overall condition, or else to treat them all. And in some people they do have all these factors and more. Although this may seem like an impossible mess to treat, it *is* possible, but needs a skilled therapist to know exactly which levels of the problem need to be worked on most to ensure the maximum healing response in minimum time.

A final "level" to look at here, is the spectre of M.E. (Myalgic Encephalomyelitis), P.V.S. (Post-Viral Syndrome) or C.F.S. (Chronic Fatigue Syndrome). This is a rather "new" arrival on the scene of possible diagnoses, not because it has only just been "created", but rather because only recently has this syndrome been researched . . . and many interesting results discovered!

Briefly, the scenario is usually one where a person becomes ill with a "virus" or a "tummy-bug". They experience the usual range of symptoms expected in these conditions, but the problem starts in the recuperative phase, ie. those with this condition don't seem to get well and recover. They may end up with a vast range of symptoms — many of them very similar to those found in Candidiasis — but specifically seem to suffer from gross, utterly debilitating exhaustion and lack of any stamina or endurance. Also, they often complain of a lot of *muscle* aches and pains — very classic of Candida too. There is more recent evidence to suggest that the Chronic Fatigue Syndrome may also be due to a cumulative toxic overload or even simply "burn-out" from chronic stress.

One differentiating point is that symptoms due to P.V.S. are inevitably made much worse by any exertion. These people have little ability to do any physical activity, and even brief bouts of such can leave them horribly depleted for days afterwards.

To date, people are told — especially by their doctors — that there is nothing that can be done, and that the problem usually resolves itself — although that could take from months to years! The reason I bring it up here is to again highlight how an apparently clear-cut case of Candidiasis may not be simply Candida. There may be many more levels to their symptom picture than at first seems apparent.

Candida they may indeed have, but often complicated by all the other above possibilities, which are not rare disease entities at all. Rather, such conditions, including P.V.S., are found commonly in our western society.

This section might best be summarised in a diagram:

BUT IS IT SIMPLY CANDIDA?

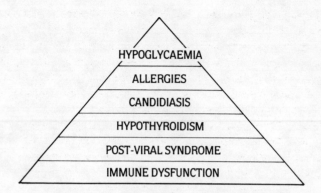

As seen from the above discussion, any or all of these levels can be found to interact, one with the other, but underneath it all lies most frequently an immune dysfunction. The overall treatment guidelines as given in this book can help enormously in restoring a person to full health again, but someone who deals with these issues on a professional basis is needed to accurately and effectively thread a way through the various possible causes, who can then formulate a highly individualised treatment program.

It is wonderful to accept responsibility for recreating health within yourself, but it is also prudent to allow yourself to be given the correct guidance to help minimise pitfalls or 'dead-end' treatments that could happen in self-diagnosis and treatment.

3 HOW CANDIDA CAN BE SPECIFICALLY DIAGNOSED

For many years, specific and accurate diagnosis of Candida was difficult. Certainly, no blood tests existed that were easy to do or reliable in results. What one was left with, as a therapist, was an understanding of Candida, and a familiarity with the symptoms that were created in someone with this condition.

Then, after learning the history of the client, it became feasible to suspect that the problems suffered by this client were due to a Candida situation. But how could this be verified? With no laboratory tests available, the only course open to follow was to put such a person on to the full Candida program. Very soon it would become apparent whether the provisional diagnosis was correct or not: if the chosen anti-fungal medication started to work, a 'die-off' reaction would occur in the first one to four weeks of therapy.

Candida in the fungal form, as it spreads throughout the body, liberates a large number of toxins. It is these toxins or poisons that are responsible for many of the symptoms Candida sufferers experience. When a substance is introduced into the body which has the ability to kill the Candida, the fungus is ruptured or destroyed and liberates massive quantities of poisons into the bloodstream. This in turn aggravates all or many of the symptoms the person with Candida experiences. This is called 'die off' where the 'dying off' of the Candida fungus results in it releasing poisons, thereby worsening — temporarily — the symptoms of a Candida sufferer.

This is an initial phase only and can be controlled in several ways. The first and most important way is to change the dose of the anti-fungal. In other words, if the fungus is breaking down too quickly because the dosage of the anti-fungal medication is too high, then *decrease* the dosage of such medicine, and within a day or so everything will settle down.

Other methods of decreasing the chances of side effects include using large amounts of Vitamin C, which helps to deactivate the toxins released, and assists the body in eliminating poisons. But by far the most effective way is to use medicinal herbs — either in tea or tincture form — to increase the eliminatory and detoxifying functions of organs such as the liver, kidneys, skin and bowels. (This will be discussed in greater detail later.)

However, back to the original issue. In the early days of Candida therapy therefore, such a "die-off" reaction experienced after starting anti-fungal medication was in fact the "test" to confirm the presence of Candida. It was often quite a dramatic "test" too, easily detected by the practitioner and certainly strongly experienced by the client, leaving little doubt that finally something WAS working.

This was particularly so, if they were one of those unfortunate people who had been through the mill with orthodoxy, constantly being told that all their tests were "normal", that in fact there was nothing physically wrong with them and therefore it all had to be in the Mind! So have a Valium or go see a psychiatrist!"

There are now at least two other ways of accurately diagnosing Candida. Although both tests have their controversial sides, the correlation between the test result and the typical scores achieved using a Candida questionnaire, are in my opinion close enough to warrant using these tests in diagnosis.

The first test, developed in the USA, is the live blood analysis test, also known as the dark-field or phase-contrast microscopy technique. Here, a small drop of blood is taken from the fingertip with a prick from a needle, and analysed using sophisticated microscopic equipment. This allows the Candida organism to be seen directly in the blood.

The second blood test involves a larger sample of blood, which is then tested for antibodies to the Candida. This test, however, needs to be done in an orthodox laboratory and requires a special request slip, ordered by a doctor. For the natural therapist, the choices of diagnosis lie within these options: (a) a thorough knowledge of client's history (incorporating the results from a comprehensive questionnaire), (b) the live blood analysis test, and (c) verification of diagnosis through the 'die off' reaction.

THE CANDIDA QUESTIONNAIRE

This questionnaire looks specifically at your symptomatology at the present time to ascertain whether there is a likelihood of a Candida infestation in your system. Carefully read through all the questions below. It is important to focus on symptoms you may be experiencing *now*, on a regular basis (daily or at least weekly). Do *not* include symptoms you may have had in the past.

SYMPTOM LEVEL	SCORE
occasional or mild	1 point
frequent or moderately severe	2 points
constant or disabling/very severe	3 points

SYMPTOMS	SCORE
Abdominal bloating.	
A lot of wind.	
Belching.	

HOW CANDIDA CAN BE SPECIFICALLY DIAGNOSED

Abdominal pain/colic.
'Irritable bowel' syndrome.
Bowel motions that are alternately too loose and then too firm (constipation).
Lethargic/tired/fatigued/feeling drained.
General muscle aches for no apparent reason.
Chronically congested/blocked nose.
Itchy eyes.
Itchy ears.
Itchy nose.
Itchy anus.
Itchy scalp.
General body feels itchy.
Muscles feel weak or paralysed.
Gums that bleed easily on brushing.
Mouth ulcers.
Gums that feel tender/sensitive/sore.
Feeling 'spacey'/disconnected from your body.
Cystitis (bladder infection), especially in females, resistant to treatment.
Poor memory.
Unable to make decisions/concentrate.
Headaches.
Migraines.
Sinusitis.
Hayfever.
Scaly scalp/dandruff.
Numbness/tingling in limbs.
Joint aches.
Nasal/throat catarrh (mucus).
Chronically sore throat.
Chronic vaginal thrush, resistant to treatment.
Pre-menstrual tension (PMT).
Menstrual problems (sore breasts/fluid retention/painful or heavy periods/irregular periods).
Eczema, resistant to treatment.
Hives.
Asthma, resistant to treatment.
Oral thrush.

UNDERSTANDING CANDIDA

Indigestion/heartburn.
Skin rashes.
Chronic 'flus'/'colds'.
Spots before the eyes.
Blurry vision.
Irritability.
Very dry mouth/lips.
Dry, scaly skin.
Scaly skin behind ears/in eyebrows/either side of the nose.
Prostatitis, resistant to treatment.
Chronic NSU (in males), resistant to treatment.
Loss of libido (sexual desire).
Anxiety spells for no reason.
Metallic taste in mouth.
Psoriasis (a scaly, reddened skin rash).
Endometriosis.
Infertile, for no apparent reason.
Impotent (unable to be sexually aroused, in males).
Vaginal itching/burning.
Allergies to yeast/mould.
Frequent mood swings.
Dizzy spells.
Allergies to foods/environmental substances.
Very sensitive to odours (perfumes, cigarette smoke, car fumes).
Bad breath.
Urgency to urinate for no apparent reason.
Chronic bronchitis.
Easily depressed, for no reason.
Feelings of 'can't cope'.
Bad body/foot odour.
Chronic ear infections.
Cracked corners of mouth.
Cravings for sugars/sweet foods/fruit/fruit juice.
Cravings for alcohol.
Cravings for bread.
Tinea of feet/groin/fingers.

HOW CANDIDA CAN BE SPECIFICALLY DIAGNOSED

Use of antibiotics (especially for acne) now or in past five years.   _____

Use of cortisone tablets/sprays/creams, now or in past 5 years.   _____

Use of the Pill, now or in past five years.   _____

Use of 'hormone replacement' for menopausal women, now or in past five years.   _____

Do damp, mouldy places make you feel worse?   _____

Do you *live* in a damp, mouldy home? YES = 3 points   _____

Have you had several, debilitating pregnancies, one after the other, in the last few years? YES = 3 points   _____

HOW YOU RATE – FEMALES:

- Less than 79 points indicates possible Candidiasis.
- Between 79 and 158 points indicates probable Candidiasis.
- Between 158 and 240 points indicates almost certain Candidiasis.

HOW YOU RATE – MALES:

- Less than 72 points indicates possible Candidiasis.
- Between 72 and 144 points indicates probable Candidiasis.
- Between 144 and 219 points indicates almost certain Candidiasis.

Questionnaires such as this one can only give an indication of the possibility of suffering from a Candida-related condition. It cannot be a definitive diagnosis. However, if after completing this exercise, the suspicion of having Candida is rather high, see a professional therapist who deals in this area of treatment to obtain validation, expert guidance and therapy.

4 NATUROPATHIC VIEWS OF WHY DISEASE OCCURS

To fully understand the approach taken by natural therapists in treating health problems, it becomes necessary to take a deeper look at the philosophical basis to our understanding of how disease occurs in the first place. This then needs to be compared with the orthodox view of how disease occurs, a concept diametrically oppposed to our perception of ill-health; one that allows for only a more restrictive way in treatment.

Ask orthodox medicine "What creates disease in general?" and the answer will be "Primarily some sort of germ." In other words, you 'catch' one or more of the thousands of different 'bugs' that always seem to be somewhere in our environment, and this creates a disease in you. That in turn leads to an approach to treatment where the most appropriate pill is found to kill that germ. Simple! Therefore, the only thing medicine needs to do is to invent better and more powerful drugs that will forever eliminate whatever germ is creating the problem — be it virus, fungus, protozoan or bacterial.

Orthodoxy has been extremely successful — on one level — in creating vast numbers of such drugs or 'magic bullets'. Although some of these chemicals indeed do have life-saving qualities, they can also have the most horrendous side-effects. The essence of most orthodox medicine is to prescribe some sort of drug that can be swallowed, applied or jabbed into you, to overcome whatever ailment you have. Generally, that is as far as it goes.

There is usually no attempt made, on broader levels, to understand *why* you have this ill-health problem in the first place. This is the vital area mostly overlooked by Western medicine, and yet it is here that the most potent answers to true healing lie.

In the above model, you need take no responsibility whatsoever for your condition. Just leave it all to your doctor. Come to them; place yourself in their hands; follow their instructions, believing that they know what's best for you and all will be well. Diet?! Mental attitudes?! Lifestyle changes?! No, don't worry about those.

"But inevitably, what happens when you take a drug, is that you allow your body to become a battle-ground between the germ and the drug. And every battlefield within which a battle is waged, ends up scarred! So too with your body. Then you need drugs for the side-effects of other drugs. Later, more drugs are taken for the side effects of the drugs used for the side effects of the original drug! Although modern medicine has saved many lives and alleviated much distress, it has also created enormous additional suffering. There are no drugs available that do not have some form of side effect, sooner or later.

So, although this approach achieves results — sometimes dramatic — the price inevitably is very high.

Natural therapy sees the issue of disease and ill-health from a different perspective, called the Vitalistic view of disease. Here, we acknowledge that germs exist, that they can create much suffering within our bodies. However, it is more than having been invaded by some bug. It is also to do with such factors as vitality, stress levels, genetic strengths or weaknesses, diet, lifestyle factors, past history of illnesses (to name but a few). The Vitalistic view of disease incorporates the concept that there is more to the body than just cells, organs, blood and bones. Whether you call it life force, vitality, good constitution, energy levels or plain old immune system doesn't really matter. The fact is that if your energy or vitality is high, and you are looking after yourself regarding diet, stress and lifestyle factors (such as smoking, drugs and alcohol), then it is less likely that you will become ill.

A classic example here is that of TB. (Even orthodox medicine will agree with this one!) People are able to pick up the germ that causes TB, but if they are really healthy, their immune system will actually create a tiny cocoon around those germs, preventing them from creating harm in the body. This especially happens if the TB germ ends up in the lung.

One can live the rest of life quite happily and healthily with those TB germs, isolated in their cysts, as long as the overall health status — or immune function — remains strong. However, if you were now to go through a series of dreadful stresses, started on the booze and drugs, and skipped meals, then you would most likely find that the cyst containing the TB germs would break down, and the disease would be activated in your system.

The factor that led to active TB in your body was not, therefore, *just* a matter of whether or not the germ was 'caught'. How your body was maintained had, in fact, a far greater influence over whether or not disease occurred. To say you caught the TB germ is too simplistic. The labels of 'TB', 'flu' or 'Candida' may be equally applied; the principles remain the same.

Viewing disease from this perspective, immediately alters the approach to it. No longer can we just consider using chemicals to 'cure' the condition. This can only get rid of the symptoms (at the risk of creating new symptoms) without getting to the root cause of the problem. Band-aid therapy, if you like.

The germ theory of disease is a narrow view that sees diseases as being caused by germs or by malfunction of a body part. If it is a germ, just throw in the drug and kill it. If it is a malfunctioning part, simply cut it out or off! Think of the

NATUROPATHIC VIEWS OF WHY DISEASE OCCURS

millions of uteri that needlessly have been taken out of women, only because there seemed to be no other way to control heavy period bleeding or cramps. Millions of tonsils because of chronic infection. Thousands of extremely expensive cardiac bypass operations or hip replacements. "You have ulcerative colitis? No worries! We'll just chop it out of you. You'll have plenty of intestines left!"

Yes, all these 'sophisticated' operations and approaches may seem to create miracles. But not once does the question arise *why* you have this problem in the first place. "What are you doing in your life that could have exacerbated this problem?" These types of questions are unpopular because they confront people with the reality that — to an enormous extent — they are responsible for what happens or doesn't happen in their bodies. It is unpopular because it entails, not guilt or blame, but an *active* participation in getting well again.

This brings up another point that further highlights the vast difference in approach taken by natural therapists. Generally, orthodox medicine accepts responsibility for getting you well again. All you need to do is to follow orders. Natural therapists say only *you* can heal yourself! A natural therapist can only act as a 'mirror' for his client, reflecting where the client may be stuck, or have strayed from the path of health. A therapist can give advice for you to follow to get well again, but only *you* can and must do the walking down the road of health. You can be supported and counselled and helped and cajoled into doing the right thing, but *you* are the one who must make the necessary changes in your diet, stress levels, lifestyle, and more.

Thus healing becomes a three-way adventure between your practitioner, yourself and your body. In most cases, health or ill-health is not just something that happens to you. Ultimately, if one wants to take this to the enth degree of esotericism, *nothing* that happens to you is ever purely by chance or co-incidence.

For now it is sufficient to just understand and be able to accept that there is more to disease than just germs or malfunction of a body part.

That there IS something extra, which in the olden days was called "Life Force" or "Vitality," but today might be expressed more scientifically as immune function or genetic constitution.

That it is the interplay of both the germ AND the Life Force that determines the final outcome as to whether disease actually eventuates or not.

That the Germ Theory of disease is primarily aimed at suppression of symptoms by the way treatment is done, whereas the Vitalistic View of disease aims treatment at deeper levels to the problem, discovered or understood by constantly asking "why is this problem in the body; what imbalances exist to allow this disease to manifest?"

UNDERSTANDING CANDIDA

The Vitalistic view of disease looks deeper into each health issue and tries to create true healing changes; this takes some time. It takes time because the body is not able to create new cells and tissues instantaneously. It may take only minutes to replace certain blood cells, but liver cells, skin cells, bone cells all have their own time-table for repair. It is thus under the action of naturopathic, healing techniques that such new cells can be generated that are far healthier than the old ones and, as this occurs, slowly but surely health returns to the ailing body.

What does all this have to do with Candida? In a case of Candida (as in any other ill-health condition too) it is *not* just a matter of swallowing some pills 'to kill it off'. Yes, this can be done, but as soon as you stop, the likelihood is extremely high that the original status of ill-health will return. You must also look at all the other factors involved, such as an important change in what you eat: your diet. Because your body has been weakened on many levels by the Candida, it now becomes essential, for full health to return, that your kidneys, bowels, liver, chest and many other glandular and organ areas are restored to full function.

When that stage is achieved then you can be considered truly cured, rather than just having had your symptoms removed. However, as this stage is not reached overnight when you use naturopathic approaches to healing, the whole process takes time: you will need patience and perseverance.

So let's take a good look at what it is we need to do, to get rid of your Candida, once and for all.

5 HOW CANDIDA *CAN* BE BEATEN

There truly is no 'magic bullet' that can be conveniently popped, killing off the Candida, leaving you with nothing else to modify in your life. It would be wonderful if this were possible, but the reality is that Candida needs to be fought on several fronts, all at once.

A mainstay to anti-Candida therapy is the yeast-free/sugar-free diet (discussed at length later in this book). Next in importance are the various substances that have powerful anti-fungal effect without destroying the friendly gut bacteria. Several years ago, the only thing really available as a natural substance was tea tree oil. Like all essential oils, this is something that needs to be treated with the utmost caution and respect as it is potentially very harmful if ingested in larger than therapeutic doses over even short periods of time. Much research has been conducted by experts, such as aroma therapists, master herbalists and the manufacturers of tea tree oil itself, as to what constitutes a safe dose. All concurred that under no circumstances should tea tree oil be taken at more than five-drop, twice daily dosages, and then only for a few months at a time. It does work in killing off Candida, both in the gut and in the general circulation, but it must be understood that this is a potentially dangerous medicine *if used internally*, and should *never* be self-prescribed. If you choose to use this substance internally as an anti-fungal, then you *must* be under the care of a professional natural therapist. I stress this issue because I know of outrageously high doses being prescribed against the advice of people who have expert knowledge of tea tree oil and its medicinal uses.

Indeed, there is absolutely no need to use tea tree oil today, as several far safer options are available. From the orthodox point of view, there are two excellent anti-fungals: Nystatin or Mycostatin, and Amphotericin or Fungilin-oral. They are remarkably safe and, if used under professional supervision, are most effective. The problem here is to find a doctor willing to prescribe the vast amounts needed for the many months it could take to treat Candida. Such doctors exist, but are few and far between. Other orthodox anti-fungals exist, such as Griseofulvin and Nizoral. The latter is particularly noxious; it has a definite potential to give you chemically induced hepatitis on top of your Candida! This one is best left alone entirely, unless every other anti-fungal has failed and serious ill-health or death is staring you in the face. Even then, you MUST be regularly monitored via blood tests to see what is happening to your liver.

Naturopathically, there are two very good, safe anti-fungals, which are extremely effective. One is Caprylic acid, derived from coconut. Since it is not absorbed from the intestinal tract, it is very safe and, despite affecting only the gut reservoir of Candida, is most effective in reducing symptoms created by this organism. It needs to be prescribed under professional supervision, and when taken must be swallowed just *before* a meal (otherwise you could end up with a nasty case of heartburn). It may also need to be taken for two to three months or longer, as decided by your therapist.

The other medicine is garlic; it has long been known to have potent anti-bacterial, anti-viral and anti-fungal properties. Laboratory studies have shown that garlic in the fresh, raw form is very effective in killing Candida. The problem for most people has been the smell! However, many deodorised brands are available on the market; the bad news is that most of them don't work very well in killing the Candida. This has been proven in laboratory tests as well as in clinical practise.

Fortunately, two companies — Nupro or Nature's Path, and Blackmores — have made a significant breakthrough in creating a garlic preparation which is relatively odourless while still retaining its anti-fungal and anti-bacterial properties, almost to the same extent as fresh, raw garlic juice. These two companies are now leading the field in providing an effective (on laboratory and clinical evidence), safe, easy-to-take anti-fungal substance. Both of these formulations are enteric-coated, ensuring that the medicine only breaks down in the small intestine. This has several advantages, not the least of which is preventing those nasty garlicky burps! Again, a professional therapist should be seen to judge what dosages or combinations are best for you.

Raw garlic is useful if taken in the diet. Onions, too, have some anti-fungal effect. It is good to cook with these two foods as frequently as possible. If you are willing to handle the stench, a fresh garlic clove can be transformed into an effective 'garlic pill' in the following way: Select a clove of garlic about the size of an average capsule. Peel it, then scratch deeply with a very sharp, pointed knife into the clove from top to bottom, all the way round. Swallow it whole. In this way the entire clove will travel through the full length of the intestines, liberating its anti-fungal effects along the way.

Some people — including some therapists — feel that as far as Candida therapy is concerned, all you need is the diet and an anti-fungal medication. If only that were so! However, with this minimal therapy you will get, in most cases, minimal results. Naturopathic approaches must always be holistic: they must take into consideration all aspects of any ill-health condition. Candida is definitely one such instance.

As well as killing off the fungus, it is vital to build up the body's life force to the point where eventually the body — hopefully by itself — will be able to maintain a healthy, balanced equilibrium between the Candida and various other gut

HOW CANDIDA CAN BE BEATEN!

inhabitants. Remember, everyone always has Candida in their gut in the *yeast* form, so to try to wipe out absolutely every last Candida germ is rather misguided. The aim is to change the Candida from the fungal form into the yeast form where, along with an ecologically balanced gut flora, and a healthy and active immune system, Candida is no longer a disease-causing factor.

To achieve this most achievable situation, the next step in the therapeutic approach is to use *acidophilus*. These are the bacteria that are used to make yoghurt, and they too are part of the bacteria that live very happily in our gut and help to maintain the balance. They do this by secreting their own anti-fungal substances.

Natural, unpasturised yoghurt supplies acidophilus, and some people with Candida are able to handle the type of protein and lactose (milk sugar) found in the yoghurt. For many others, yoghurt, despite its valuable source of acidophilus, creates a multitude of miseries, either by inducing allergic or food sensitivity reactions or by fostering further Candida growth through the lactose. If this is the case, cut yoghurt out of the diet.

Whether you are able to handle yoghurt or not, it is highly advisable to take a potent supplement of acidophilus. Many different formulations exist on the market. Virtually all of these have one problem in common: the tablet or capsule dissolves in the stomach. The acidophilus powder is even more of a problem because, when the acidophilus comes in contact with stomach acids, a huge proportion — some experts claim as much as 90 per cent — of this acidophilus is destroyed before it gets to the small intestines, and lower in the gut where it is most needed. It is a common fallacy that because acidophilus creates an acidic environment, it can handle the extremely potent stomach acids. This is not so.

To overcome this situation, Nature's Path has put out a capsule of acidophilus called Biodophilus. Its great advantage is that it has an acid-resistant coating on it, and cannot dissolve in the very acidic environment of the stomach. Once in the alkaline area of the small intestine, it is able to dissolve, liberating the full bolus of the concentrated, live acidophilus. Because of its potency and its method of specific delivery, a far smaller amount of Biodophilus is needed than would be required from other products on the market.

Candida can and does have a serious effect on more than just the gut itself. Various organs such as the brain, heart, liver, kidneys as well as the thyroid and uterus, bladder and lungs are all affected and weakened. By simply remaining on the anti-Candida diet and killing off the Candida, the body will heal itself again, with time. But this can take many, many months to many years, if the body is left alone to its own, weakened devices.

Yet, given some support, the body has remarkable recuperative and healing powers, but these need to be helped along. Here, potent medicinal herbs are extremely valuable and should always be prescribed in any case of Candida. The ultimate aim is not just to kill off the Candida, but to strengthen the entire system, so that at the end of treatment the body is so restored to normal function that it needs no supports at all. Like a broken leg, when the bone eventually is healed, the cast is taken off.

The simple herbal teas such as rosehip, chamomile and peppermint are good and pleasant to take. But they are not strong enough in the type of medicinal action that is needed to restore normal function to a Candida-ravished body. Medicinal herbs are prescribed in various ways, either as capsules, pills, tinctures or teas. The tinctures contain some alcohol, which is normally forbidden on any Candida regime. However, by clinical trial and error, it has been my experience that the majority of people can handle this small amount of alcohol with no problems whatsoever. Then there is a small proportion of people with Candida who can't, and when they take it they can react quite violently. For these people, an alternative way of prescribing medicinal herbs becomes imperative, because it is they who need the healing action of herbs the most.

There seem to be no readily available herbal capsules that have the right combination of herbs that not only stimulate the immune system, but also give healing support to the weakened areas. It became necessary to formulate my own herbal tea mix, one that could be tolerated by both sensitive and stronger people and covered all the major body areas (the intestines, thyroid, kidneys, lymphatics, liver, immune system, pancreas, stomach, brain, thymus gland, nervous system). Most importantly, it had to be not too vile to drink!

This tea now exists as the C-Herb Tea (C for Candida). It is extremely potent and, like all medicine, needs to be started with a small dose and then slowly increased, as tolerated. If the tea were to be increased too fast, you could end up with some nausea, irritability, tiredness or a nasty headache. None of these symptoms are dangerous or long lasting, once the dose is stopped or reduced. Certainly the effect is unpleasant, due to the body being pushed too rapidly into a healing and cleansing mode. (Just as a very, very dusty room is best cleaned gently, rather than rushing madly in, waving your feather duster around, putting the fan on, and then choking on the dust thus aroused, so too it is in cleansing your body inside.)

These medicinal herbs work in several ways. The Candida produces a vast number of very poisonous substances — hence all the symptoms. These poisons weaken the body, including the major organs of elimination such as the liver, kidneys, bowel, skin and lungs. With time, the body becomes less and less able to detoxify or clean itself, resulting in a vicious cycle of further poisoning and further weakening of these organs of cleansing.

This cycle must (and can) be broken to restore normal function, increasing your sense of well-being. These herbs, especially by improving the liver and kidney function, also increase the rate at which the vast amounts of toxins released initially in Candida therapy — the 'die off' reaction — can be eliminated. If all these factors are carefully taken into account and the right combination of medicinal substances prescribed, die-off should become, and does become, far less of an issue than if just left to the body's own weakened devices.

These medicinal herbs work, not only by increasing organ or glandular function, but by allowing those weakened areas to repair themselves. Once again, the emphasis in this approach to Candida is not on 'kill and leave' (killing the fungus, then leaving the body to itself), unrealistically expecting your body to be now totally okay. In a few cases this will be so. In the majority of cases, much support and healing is needed.

This C-Herb Tea formula contains these herbs:

Agrimony	1 part
Bladderwrack	1 part
Clivers	1 part
Dandelion root	1 part
Echinacea	1 part
Fennel	¼ part
Globe Artichoke	1 part
Meadowsweet	1 part
Rosemary	½ part
Thyme	⅕ part
Vervain	½ part
White poplar	½ part
Yarrow	1 part
Borage	1 part

These herbs are specially blended and milled to a specific consistency or fineness, and then made precisely as directed. The non-practitioner who attempts this formula will encounter many difficulties. Firstly, the average health food store does not stock many of these medicinal herbs. Secondly, the major suppliers of such herbs only sell in bulk. Thirdly, the herbs are sold in a very coarse state and need to be specially milled for maximum effect. It is very important that the herbs are in fact the botanically correct ones and that they are always of a very high quality. Old, mouldy herbs are obviously *not* an advantage in Candida therapy, but if the proper quality is obtained, they become an invaluable and indeed essential component.

Lastly, this herb tea needs to be made in a definite way. It needs to stand for several hours to allow the active ingredients to fully draw out into the solution (it is recommended that the tea be made the night before). When it is ready, simply stir the tea, strain off the required dose and reheat to very hot — but not boiling. The dose should be taken two to five times a day, as tolerated. The herbs work better on an empty stomach, but if this is too uncomfortable or strong, then have some food shortly afterwards.

If you find it inconvenient or difficult to brew or reheat the tea for your lunchtime dose, then take it in a thermos. Several days' worth of tea can be made at a time and left in the fridge for up to about four days. The ratio of mix is one teaspoon of tea for each cup and, although you should start on only quarter of a cup at a time, eventually your body will tolerate the full dose. The tea should *never* be made in an aluminium or cast-iron container (glass, enamel, stainless steel or pottery is fine).

Diet, anti-fungals, bacterial replacement and support to the general body through potent, healing, medicinal herbs constitute the essentials in Candida therapy. Many additional techniques and supplements exist to further the healing process. Some practitioners would argue that a few — or perhaps most — of these extras are (to them) essential, but here you could end up with one big problem: overkill. You would have so many pills and potions to take, so many things to do, that Candida therapy would become a complicated nightmare of extraordinary expense.

Nevertheless, let's take a look at some of these other options, all very valid in themselves, but ones which I regard as extras rather than as essentials, in my view of Candida therapy.

6 EXTRA DIMENSIONS TO CANDIDA THERAPY

As a herbalist, my approach to treating Candida would obviously lean towards using medicinal herbs as a major component of therapy aimed at restoring full, balanced function to the body in a holistic way. However, there are many ways of achieving an end result. Acupuncture, homeopathy, counselling, rebirthing, vitamin therapy or any number of others also have their part to play in Candida therapy. Being the eclectic person I am, I have no hesitation in using other tools to fight this potentially resistant and dangerous fungus.

I firmly believe that there is much need for vitamin supplementation. Many people object to this, saying that we should be able to derive all the vitamins we need from our diet. Indeed, this is true — theoretically. Think for a moment about how our food is grown, stored and then eaten. Firstly, our soils are notoriously depleted of various nutrients and our food consequently lacking, despite the use of artificial fertilisers. Then the food becomes filled with spray residues and it is impossible to eliminate these entirely despite washing or peeling. A great deal of our food is picked unripe, and then artificially ripened (just think of the tomatoes you are so often forced to buy), placed into cold storage for long periods and finally, transported over vast distances to other coolrooms, this time at your greengrocer. Then, time on the display shelves, time in your fridge and usually too much time in the cooking pot. Not much of the original vitamin content is left by the time you put that food into your mouth.

That isn't the end of the story: it gets worse. Most of us, and especially those who have Candida, have poor digestive systems which are unable to efficiently extract goodness from our food (whatever goodness is still left). As we *all* live under stress, our requirements for vitamins and minerals are very high. The final conclusion: vitamin and mineral supplementation is very important, especially for people with Candida.

This raises a different issue. Megadoses of vitamins seems to be the 'in' fad at the moment, although some of the more recent literature is indicating that perhaps some of those megadoses need to be reassessed. Individually, there are a vast number of vitamins that could be prescribed for Candida treatment. If these were to be used in megadoses — which is not really applicable or necessary for everyone — then you would end up with an enormous number of pills to swallow. As Candida therapy is not over and done with in simply a few weeks, it is not a course I would advise to follow.

I have had clients who came in and when we got to the section of the consultation where I ask what medications they are taking, I end up with half my desk literally covered with a multitude of pills and potions. It's interesting that we as Natural Therapists tend to point the finger at orthodoxy about *their* pill-popping ventures! I feel that for some in the so called "natural" field of healing, there needs to be a closer and more realistic evaluation of our own situation, before the finger is pointed so self-righteously.

The issue is NOT whether all these vitamins and supplements work or not. I firmly believe they do. However, the issue is more "can our clients realistically afford all these vast numbers of pills, and in fact, are they ALL essential?" It is distressing to see again and again clients who feel they have to spend $80 to $150 per week on medicines. There are just too many people who cannot afford such medical bills — besides consultation costs! — and it IS up to us as practitioners to ensure that we do some deep thinking and come up with an overall therapeutic regime that will work ... and is affordable! Or is Candida therapy to sink to the status of an elitist treatment ie. only those with "big bucks" can afford to get well?

The following recommendations are not the only ones that can be prescribed. However, they are the ones I've had good results with. They are also economical, in that the one tablet contains a wide variety of nutrients that improve overall body function. So less pill-popping and less dollars. If you do decide to remain on other varieties of supplements, then always make sure they are yeast-free and sugar-free, and that the formulations are properly balanced. (This is especially important with the B-group formulations. Here, if all the primary Bs — B_1, B_2, B_3, B_5 and B_6 are provided in equal proportions, then this is unbalanced and can create or exacerbate imbalances within your body.) Hiltons* is a company that supplies an excellent range of supplements and the advantage is that they are easy to obtain anywhere in Australia. All you need to do is lift your phone receiver and within a few days the medicines arrive by post. Their formula 127 is an excellent all-round medicine, providing multivitamins, minerals, B-complex (balanced), enzymes, amino acids and some herbs. The dosage should range from 1 to 3 tablets a day (as with all doses given here, they can only be a guide. A professional therapist who knows about these issues will prescribe the precise amounts that you need, based on your particular problem, constitution, toxic status and so much more).

Many people with Candida suffer terribly from lethargy, and a remarkably useful substance here is Coenzyme Q_{10}. This acts powerfully in many ways, but,

---

* If this formula is not available in your country, then try to get a formula with the same or similar contents — see appendix.

especially, it improves energy status and strengthens the immune system. This enhances the body's own capacity to fight and control Candida. Dosage ranges from 2 to 6 capsules a day. Many producers market this product, but not all of them work as well as they should. My experience, backed up by the research literature on CoQ_{10} over the years, indicates that CoQ_{10} in the oil form works best, rather than the dry, powdered form.

Vitamin C is a wonderful, all-round vitamin to use in virtually any ill-health problem, certainly in Candida. It is one of the few vitamins where I have almost no reservations about it being used in vast quantities, subject only to bowel tolerance. However, this should be guided by a practitioner. Many different brands exist, but it is important to get one that is free of all yeast, colouring, flavouring and sugar. The powdered form is probably the most economical way to use it if large doses are prescribed. This is one vitamin that I feel should be used in greater quantities than is found in most multivitamin formulations.

There are many people with Candida who suffer from a lack of hydrochloric acid production in their stomachs. Not only does this result in poor digestion and a greater tendency towards food allergies, it also allows the Candida to survive more easily in the gut. Nature's Own makes a good product here called Hydrochloric Acid — Plus* and one tablet should be taken with each meal, or as directed by your therapist. Other good products exist, but check that none of their components is yeast-derived.

Essential fatty acids are important for immune function too, and here GLA or Evening Primrose oil can be of use. However, they are extraordinarily expensive and there is also research evidence that claims they can have an immune depressive effect if too much is taken. For these reasons, I prefer to obtain the essential fatty acids from safflower oil, which can be combined with olive oil (both in the cold-pressed form). Mix them half and half and use as often as possible in your cooking and for salad dressings. It can even be taken neat every day (one to six teaspoons), and has the advantage of reducing hunger pangs in a very safe and effective way, when taken with meals.

Many people with Candida suffer from allergic reaction to foods. To decrease the symptoms of such reactions, you can very safely use — and self-prescribe — the tissue salt Nat. phos. 6X. This medicine is taken in the mouth, 1 to 2 tablets at a time, and allowed to dissolve. Do not swallow, as this nullifies any therapeutic effect. This medicine helps to decrease body acidity and, via this mechanism,

---

* If this formulation is not available in your country, then try to get a formula with the same or similar contents (see Appendix).

decreases symptoms created by food reactions. Another way in which such an effect can be obtained is by adding 1 tsp. of Alfalfa seed to every 3 cups of C-Herb Tea, when preparing the tea. The dose of the Nat. phos. 6X can be repeated several times, every five to ten minutes as needed. Most cases respond extremely well to this simple medicine, despite the fact the tiny pills contain lactose. If you get a reaction, then stop taking them.

Wheat grass juice is often touted as a cure-all. It certainly is a very good and effective supplement that can be added to any Candida program. Again, the cost might be daunting, as the dried product, whether of barley juice or wheat juice, is extremely expensive. With a little bit of effort, you can easily grow wheat grass and juice it yourself. You need only your two jaws and a good set of teeth — false or natural! Simply buy organic wheat from the health food store (not from produce stores, as it could be sprayed with potentially deadly chemicals). Get a flat tray about 6 to 8cm deep and fill it with some good soil. Soak enough of the whole wheat to entirely cover the soil. Let it soak overnight and then sow on top of the soil. Cover with Gladwrap or a damp cloth, and place in a warm, dark space for 2 to 4 days. The soil must be moist, but not wet. As soon as the grain starts to sprout, bring it into the light. After a day or so, put it in a sunny position and keep the soil moist. Once the grass is approximately 20cm tall, harvest as much as will fit between your thumb and middle finger by cutting the grass as close to the soil as possible. Rinse well, shake dry and chew. Swallow the juice and spit out the residue. If the taste is too strong, sip some water as you chew. You can safely do this once or twice a day. A veritable 'living' multivitamin/multimineral medicine!

Homeopathy provides some very valuable tools for treating Candida too, but it is my experience and that of a lot of clients who had already tried Homeopathy before they came to see me, that although it certainly can improve a lot of symptoms created by Candida and slowly improve the overall status of the body, nevertheless, some extra medicines will be needed too. The diet always remains very important, as does the use of anti-fungals, plus Acidophilus supplementation. However, it seems that if homeopathy is used when a person is riddled with Candida and before the reservoirs of this noxious organism are decreased — especially in the gut — the treatment can result in violent reactions to the homeopathic medicines.

Hence, I always use the regimes described in this book to decrease the Candida numbers first, and then I use homeopathy if necessary. One area in which homeopathy is excellent is in providing a Candida nosode. This can greatly reduce Candida-related symptoms, but, again, is not to be used in the initial period of treatment. This nosode is a highly diluted preparation of the Candida organism itself and is administered under the tongue. It seems to work very much like the

EXTRA DIMENSIONS TO CANDIDA THERAPY

Candida vaccines that some researchers refer to in their literature, but has the advantage that it does not need to be injected as the vaccine does. So people are more able to self-administer it as needed. It is especially useful in desensitising a person with Candida to mouldy, yeasty or fermented products, and is excellent when used in the later stages of treatment.

Acupuncture also can play an important role in healing people with Candida. This can be used simultaneously with any of the treatments outlined in this book and would be highly beneficial and is recommended, if economically viable.

Exercise is another aspect that should be looked at in a balanced way. Most people suffering with Candida are already in an exhausted state, and those with any post-viral syndrome component to their problem will not be able to spare any energy at all, let alone for exercise. It is true that the body needs exercise; people with any ill-health problem, especially the type discussed here, should exercise, but *only* as their body allows them.

As you get better and stronger, the spare energy will be there to use. There is of course the potential malingerer who will hide behind the 'I'm-too-tired' excuse, but anyone who really wants to get well, and with even a bit of commonsense and honest self-appraisal, will know when their bodies are ready to be exercised.

Start with perhaps gentle walking and build up as tolerated to any form of exercise that suits you. There is no point in choosing an exercise that may be excellent, but one which you hate and are more likely to drop than continue.

Stress is the great saboteur of any illness or any treatment regime. In our Western lives, it is an unavoidable issue and must be confronted. There are people who do all the right things, yet respond only very slowly. When their situation is looked at more closely, it can be seen that they are under a lot of stress, at home, at work or wherever, and this literally sabotages their progress. It is not until the stress is more effectively dealt with that real results in healing can be seen.

There are a vast number of ways to reduce stress, but one I wish to review is the alpha/theta meditation cassette.* Meditation does many things, one of which is to put us into an alpha or theta state of brainwave activity (relaxation and deep relaxation respectively). Here finally, is a scientific and extremely easy way to induce relaxation at will. All that is needed is a cassette recorder (preferably a walkman, but not essential), a quiet area in which you will not be disturbed, and the will to be relaxed. Depending on how deeply relaxed you want to become, listen to either the alpha or theta side of the cassette, on a very low

---

* See Appendix for further information.

volume so that you can just hear the bipping sound. Allow yourself to flow with the sound and within minutes you should feel yourself relax. This process can be heightened by consciously relaxing every part of your body, starting with your toes and ending with the top of your scalp. It is in this deep state of relaxation that the body may strengthen and reconstruct itself.

This is only the beginning! Although this is a whole subject in itself, just briefly, it is good to know that you can use your mind power to heal yourself faster and more effectively. This process is called creative visualisation (a good book to read on this topic is called *Creative Visualisation* by Shakti Gawain*). It is while you are in a state of alpha or theta that you are able to more powerfully use creative visualisation. Although this is getting into the Metaphysical areas of Healing and may be too fringe for some, nevertheless it is ultimately the true Source of all Healing, and from this perspective, the above cassette plus Gawain's book are highly recommended as a potent, scientific way of enhancing your recovery from Candida or any other illness.

THE CANDIDA PROGRAM SO FAR:

- The anti-Candida, yeast-free/sugar-free diet.
- Anti-fungals (such as Nupro's Entrogar, also known as Nature's Path Garlicin; Blackmore's Garlix, and Caprylic acid).
- Acidophilus gut replacement (via Nature's Path Biodophilus).
- Holistic body regeneration (via the C-Herb Tea).
- Supplements (such as Hiltons product no. 127, and Natures Own Hydrochloric Acid — Plus).

This already constitutes a fair number of pills and potions to take, but it is seen as the core of my approach to Candida therapy, and will definitely work in controlling and overcoming a condition of gastrointestinal or systemic Candidiasis.

Extras would include:

- Coenzyme Q_{10}.
- Vitamin C.
- Nat. phos. 6X (a tissue salt).
- Wheat grass juice.

* See Appendix for further information.

EXTRA DIMENSIONS TO CANDIDA THERAPY

- Cold-pressed safflower/olive oil.
- Homeopathic Candida nosode.
- Acupuncture.
- Stress reduction (including metaphysical approaches to healing).
- Exercise program.

A major problem in many Candida treatment programs is a state of 'overkill' with the range of 'tools' used. Although all may be valid on one level, realism dictates that one must choose wisely from the many to reach a combination of the ESSENTIAL few.

7 WHEN I'M WELL AGAIN . . .

You've been diagnosed as having Candida, you have been placed on the anti-Candida program; what else do you need to know? Die-off as discussed earlier, is important to understand; if you don't, you may feel that the treatment is not working. This phenomena can begin on the first day of treatment in some sensitive people, or after several weeks on the program.

It may also return many weeks later, when you seem to be really improving and feeling great again. Out of the blue, you could have a sudden flare-up of old symptoms. The most likely cause is another bout of die-off, unless you have strayed from the program (then this will be the cause of your suffering). Decrease your dose of anti-fungal medication and within a few days you should be getting over it. Extra Vitamin C and the C-Herb Tea can help to mitigate the severity of the symptoms at this time.

If things have not settled down within seven days, perhaps you're not dealing with a die-off at all. It now becomes essential to contact your practitioner and have your situation thoroughly checked out.

One final point about die-off. It often has all the classic symptoms of flu, such as runny nose, thick head, fuzzy mind, congested sinuses, earaches, even fever. At this point, some clients panic and rush to the doctor, only to be prescribed . . . antibiotics.

Firstly, most flus (if this IS a flu) are caused by viruses. Antibiotics CANNOT kill viruses, so all that happens is that you encourage your Candida even more. Antibiotics are not only toxic, but will also depress an already faltering immune system. However, antibiotics DO have a place in life-threatening situations. If you're not sure as to whether you are experiencing die-off or whether you do in fact have a dose of the flu, then contact your practitioner for further advice and take the following steps.

There is a very old herbal formula that is immensely effective either in preventing a flu from developing if taken early enough, or in shortening the duration of a flu if it is already established. If it is only die-off no harm will come from doing the following: Buy equal amounts of Yarrow, Elderflower and peppermint teas. Mix together thoroughly and store in an airtight container, opaque to light. This can be labelled as your 'flu tea'. Prepare by pouring one cup of boiling water over one heaped teaspoon of the mix and allow to steep for at least 20 minutes. Reheat, strain and drink copious quantities (3 to 8 cups a day).

This helps to increase the Life Force/Vitality and allows the body to fight any bug like a virus. For extra zap, a small piece of fresh ginger root, the size of half a thumb, could be chopped very finely and added to the brew. Rest, keep up the

UNDERSTANDING CANDIDA

fluids, decrease your food intake and before long — if it is the flu — you should be well again.

This regime can be further strengthened by taking copious amounts of Vitamin C, plus some extra Vitamin A (the beta-carotene form is best here) in doses not exceeding 20 000iu per day, for adults. Garlic would normally be prescribed for any flu, but as you may be uncertain if this is die-off or flu, then it is best to at least initially ease off or stop any garlic medicine you may be taking as your anti-fungal. If it turns out that you do have the flu, then by all means resume the garlic treatment.

One seemingly contradictory phenomenon that can happen in Candida therapy is an increased sensitivity to certain foods *after* having been on the treatment for some time. If people break their diet they find that foods or beverages that they once could handle now cause rather drastic reactions. It puzzles people: they assumed the reaction would be less, not greater, if they are supposed to be getting better.

Several issues are involved here. Firstly, imagine what it would have been like if you had had 6 to 10 cups of coffee, or 20 to 30 cigarettes a day. On a day-to-day basis, although somewhere deep down you would have known it wasn't doing you any good, on superficial levels you would have seemed to have handled the caffeine or nicotine quite well.

Then, if you had gone cold turkey, you would have realised how much effect those seemingly innocuous substances had had on your body. After the withdrawal phase, if you then decided to have a cup of coffee or a cigarette, what would have happened? With the coffee you would have become all hyper and jittery, while with the cigarette you would have felt an initial sense of dizziness and nausea again, due to the nicotine.

Once your body has had a rest from such poisons and has lost the built-up tolerance to them, it is sensitive once more, and it lets you know in no uncertain terms how poisonous caffeine and nicotine really are to your body.

The same type of situation happens if you have unsuspected food allergies or sensitivities. If you have been taking them day in, day out, to an extent your system has built up a tolerance to them. Once the body has been given a break and has re-sensitised, when those types of foods are reintroduced — especially when breaking the diet — your body can react quite violently.

Another level to this problem is that Candida toxins are known to paralyse your immune system. It is primarily through your immune system that you react to certain substances. When you are in a state of full-blown Candida, your 'reaction system' (the immune system) is literally turned off, and therefore unable to react.

WHEN I AM WELL AGAIN...

When you start treatment and remove many of these reactive substances from your diet, you finally give your immune system a chance to get up off the floor, as it were, to dust itself off and fight back. Secondly, as the Candida is killed off, less of the fungus remains to produce poisons that can paralyse your immune system; once again the immune response is able to reassert itself. If a potentially allergenic substance is reintroduced into your body, you will get a reaction because the system is now able to fight back.

This is only a temporary phase, one that may last several months, but eventually your body repairs itself so well — especially through the use of the herbs in the C-Herb Tea — that the body is able to ingest even foods that previously were a problem. At this stage real healing has taken place.

Overall length of treatment varies depending on many different factors, such as the extent of Candida infestation, constitutional strength, type of healing program adhered to, previous length of infection, and many more. The above-average case of Candida, but with good constitutional capacity for healing and very hard work with the program, can expect to see promising results within three to four months.

The average case could take six to eight months to really clear up and heal and some people, again for a wide variety of reasons, could take much longer to overcome the fungus. However, they are in the minority. Once the symptoms have cleared up and you are feeling well again, then you can afford to be more lenient with the diet but do so with great care! At this stage it is vital to consolidate your progress for a few months. If a cast is taken off a broken leg that has only just started to mend, the chances are great that it will break again. If it had been left on for just a little longer time, the bone would have been allowed to really strengthen. So too with your body, which may have been horribly depleted and affected by the Candida. Don't be too eager to drop the treatment altogether, too soon. You could waste all the effort and time — not to mention the money — you have already invested.

In this time of consolidation, remain primarily on the diet. Continue with at least a minimum of anti-fungal medication, with a minimum of Biodophilus and preferably one to three cups of the C-Herb Tea a day. One tablet of the Hiltons 127 a day would not go astray either.

When your healing has been truly consolidated (after one to three months of the reduced regime), there is a choice. It would be most appropriate to seek professional advice to find what would be best for you. If you only had a light degree of Candida to begin with, perhaps you could now stop all medications, although it would be foolish to go back on to yeasts, mouldy, fermented or sugary foods or beverages at this stage.

Once every four to six months for the next one to two years, it would be wise to take a course of an anti-fungal medication, plus some Biodophilus and C-Herb Tea, only for a month or so, in case the gut ecology is getting out of balance again. Once you have had full-blown Candida, for several years at least, if not longer, you may be susceptible to a relapse, depending on what you do to yourself.

Simply as a form of insurance, it is advisable for those who have had severe Candidiasis, once they are completely well again, to remain on a minimum of the following treatments:

- C-Herb Tea, daily.
- Biodophilus, 1 capsule a day.
- Hiltons product no. 127, 1 tablet a day.

Such a long-term insurance program costs very little in time and money and is a small price to pay for continued good health and well-being.

SECTION II

Detailed Explanation of the Candida Diet

1 RESPONSIBILITY AND HEALING: INSEPARABLE COMPANIONS

Many people complain that the Candida diet is 'too much work'. If you're the average sort of Westerner, your habit of food preparation and eating is probably an important reason why you are not in your present ill-health predicament. Is there anything in this life that ultimately doesn't have to be worked for?

The reality is that everything we do needs an energy expenditure of some sort. It is also true that often you can invest a minimum of energy into something — like breakfast or lunch — and seem to get away with it . . . for a while! Eventually however, you pay the price for those skipped or hastily gulped down meals. It doesn't happen immediately and, in a sense, that is unfortunate! If the results were more direct, you would clearly see the correlation and might be more likely to do things in a less destructive way. The problem is that the human body is remarkably versatile, adaptable and resilient. But even this magnificent machine of ours eventually reaches a breaking point. When the events leading up to such a breakdown have become the 'normal' way of life over a long period of time, it is hard to see the connection. Then, if this is pointed out, people baulk at the facts, with excuses: "But I haven't got the time", "I've got to get the kids off to school . . .".

The ultimate question is do you *truly* want to get well, or do you want to *play* at getting well? If it is the former, then be realistic and prepare to make changes in your life; that is the only way things will improve. It's the old adage of 'what you put in is what you get out'!

It is the change-over period from one way of life to another, more constructive way that is the hardest time. Once you have settled into a new pattern, you'll wonder what all the fuss was about! It doesn't take years: usually one to two short months or so and these types of changes are set.

The concept of working hard for our boss, saving for a holiday, or digging in the garden is not difficult for us to understand and accept. But the very thought of *working* to become healthy seems unreal; we have been trained in the concept of the "magic bullet" approach to illness which involves no work beyond simply swallowing a pill.

Health doesn't just happen to most of us. To obtain a good level of health *and to maintain it* requires work. The sooner that is faced, the easier the whole thing becomes.

2 THE ANTI-CANDIDA DIET: A BASIS TO YOUR THERAPY

Nutrition and diet can be frustrating aspects of natural therapy. Every 'authority' on diet seems to have their own view, often fully 'supported' by all manner of trials and scientific data. Yet, when you look at even a few of these diets, they seem to conflict, often on some serious points. So, who *is* correct? It's a nightmare for practitioners to sort out; for the average person-on-the-street it seems impossible.

Well, even as a therapist, I found myself caught up in all the arguments and counter-arguments, as well as volumes upon volumes of data, all supposed to support, but ultimately only to confuse the entire issue. So back to square one; what would a person eat in the wild, away from the technological processing of food? You would obviously eat whatever Nature — in her wisdom — had provided for you: fish, fowl (of all sorts), eggs, raw milk, nuts, honey, tubers, seeds, grains, fruit, vegetables, and more. What then of food combining? A healthy body should be able to handle *any* combination of food at the same time whether it is a 'good' one or not.

However, who in reality is so entirely healthy that they are able to handle *any* combination of foods? This is when you should listen — not to authoritative people, books or studies — but to *your* body! It will tell you without a shadow of doubt if it can't handle certain types of foods or combinations. For some it will require becoming more sensitively attuned to what their bodies are telling them; this is not impossible to achieve.

What about milk, fruit and honey? They are provided by Nature. Why are they excluded from the Candida diet? There are good reasons, in my experience. Firstly, let's address the problems with milk products such as yoghurt, buttermilk, cream and various cheeses.

An enormous number of people in our society are allergic to dairy foods. This is usually in reaction to the lactose in the milk, either directly because their bodies can't handle it, or indirectly because lactose, being a sugar, stimulates Candida growth in the gut. Many people also react to the specific protein of milk, as well as to the lactose content.

Yoghurt is a big problem for people with especially severe Candida. This often surprises, as the Acidophilus in the yoghurt is supposed to not only supply this much needed bacteria to the gut of a person with Candida, but the very chemical composition of the protein in the yoghurt is supposed to be changed by this bacterium to a more acceptable and digestible form for the body. Nevertheless, it is not until they finally eliminate it from their diet that real progress starts to be made on the road to better health.

That leaves fruit, fruit juice and honey to be explained. None of these foods is inherently bad, except if you happen to have Candida. *Any* sugar feeds Candida! That's the bottom line. Fruit, especially fruit juice (yes, even the one with 'no added sugar'), is loaded with sugar. Natural sugar no doubt, but still sugar! (Ah, but then carrot juice must be okay because it is a vegetable. Unfortunately, carrots are LOADED with sucrose: a sugar.) Indeed, it is full of all sorts of other "goodies" too, especially beta carotene, which will help heal your bowel wall lining, but the amount of sucrose and its Candida-feeding ability, simply cancels out any therapeutic effect. Sorry but therefore even carrot juice is definitely out!

Do I need to explain why honey too is definitely *off* the list? *Absolutely all sugars are out!*

As the Candida diet is a basic component of any anti-Candida therapy and needs to be maintained for a long time, it is vital that the diet is well balanced and nourishing. Too many Candida diets exist that create significant malnourishment even over just a few months. The Candida diet is not just a diet, it is a way of life. It is essential that all the primary food groups are represented (protein, carbohydrate, fats and oil, vegetables and, eventually, fruit). Often, people become very concerned that fruit is taken from the diet, thinking that they will suffer from lack of vitamins and minerals. Fruit however, is withdrawn for only the initial four to eight weeks of therapy; besides, vergetables contain more than enough of these nutrients.

It is important that the diet is as non-fanatical as possible. Provide as open an arena of food possibilities, while still allowing for the control and healing of Candidiasis. Only a few very ill and sensitive Candida clients really need to be on the very restricted version. There cannot be a 'standard' diet. People are too variable for such a thing to be practical.

Basic guidelines are needed, but within these parameters it is important for each individual to find out for themselves what it is that they can or cannot handle. It is important to restrict two basic components: yeast and sugars. If in this diet it says it is okay to have, for example, wheat, but you are allergic to it, then listen to your body, not to me. This is where the concept of a food diary comes in.

To accurately isolate which foods may be giving you problems, for two to three weeks, write down everything you eat. Record the time of your meal/snack, then note how you are feeling; for example, sleepy, spaced out, achy, terrific. Next, list everything that was in the meal; for example, bread (yeast free), butter, avocado, salt, lettuce.

Over a period of two or three weeks, you will find correlations between how you felt and what you had been eating. When a food is highlighted by this method, test it.

Choose a time when you are feeling well (very masochistic!), then 'challenge' yourself with that particular food, by eating a lot of it. Observe what happens. From the next few minutes to hours if you start to experience symptoms, your suspicions will be confirmed. Put such foods on the 'no' list. It is easy to forget the reaction, as time goes by, especially if there are a lot of foods you are reacting to.

Although this process is a bit tedious, it can uncover some interesting information and is well worth the effort for those few weeks. Blood tests can be done to uncover allergies, but many can be unreliable, alternately giving a false positive or a false negative result, confusing the whole issue.

What to do if you are suffering from vast numbers of allergies or food sensitivities? If all the foods that affected you were removed from the diet, malnourishment could eventuate. These allergies, to an enormous extent, are due to the Candida in the first place. As this is treated and as the body is restored to normal function by the use of powerful, medicinal herbs or supplements, such allergic or food-sensitivity responses will diminish and, finally, disappear. Remove the worst of the reaction-causing foods and rotate the remaining ones as much as possible. With time, as the body strengthens, the offending items can be carefully reintroduced.

For many people, the Candida diet is extremely confronting. Suddenly they are deprived of many of the 'nice' things in their life: coffee, tea, alcohol, cigarettes, sugars. These items are only luxuries in our life, but, because of the way we Westerners live in today's world, these are often not seen as luxuries, but as necessities. However, it is clear that they are not nutritious at all; conversely, they harm the body, over time. They are not essentials for maintaining a healthy body.

Candida or no Candida, these type of items should definitely be quite restricted or eliminated from our diet anyway. This is why the Candida diet, as outlined here is so healthy for you. It is balanced in all the food groups and is not fanatical. It does take away several types of substances usually seen as "normal" foods — but that is in fact an advantage to you.

The important thing to realise for someone who has Candida is simply this. You are already ill and feeling unwell. A major reason for such feelings is the type of diet you are now on (including the so-called "pleasurable" items.) But it is definitely these very "pleasurable" substances that are creating so much of your misery!

The answer is to cut these out — not necessarily easy to do, admittedly. But what other choice is there in fact? Taking anti-fungals alone is not enough. The diet IS an essential component of the overall therapy. The sooner this reality is faced and constructive action taken, the sooner you will start to experience what REAL health is all about. The choice is yours.

You can keep going on and off the diet, but you will also not get very far in the healing process. As with giving up smoking, there just comes the time when a decision has to be made and stuck with.

The problems begin if, besides giving up the yeasty, fermented foods and the sugars, you are also addicted to coffee, tea, alcohol and cigarettes. Then you have some *work* ahead. Decide which one of these would be the least difficult to give up and focus on it. Set yourself a goal and a time limit, and go for it. There will be occasions when you break from the diet. That's only human: don't get caught up in guilt or blame as they are useless and destructive energies. Just acknowledge that you could have made a more constructive choice; realise that this program is for your own good, and then get back into it again. Don't give up entirely – like some of my clients tried to do, simply because they broke the diet once or twice. That certainly is throwing the baby out with the bath water!

Realise that every step you take in the right direction is far, far better than just standing on the spot doing nothing. Be absolutely firm with yourself and keep pushing yourself, but ironically perhaps, also be willing to have a sense of gentleness about it all. Do the best you can and realise that success breeds further success. Stick with your commitment!

This diet will normalise your weight: if you are overweight, you will lose weight, if you are underweight, you should gain. An extremely serious problem connected with a few other so-called Candida diets is that people who cannot afford to lose weight, do so. This is usually the result of fanatically restrictive food lists, providing unbalanced nutrition. IF YOU LOSE BODY WEIGHT YOU CAN'T AFFORD TO LOSE ON THE DIET OUTLINED IN THIS BOOK, *YOU ARE DOING IT WRONG*. This can be stated so strongly because of the many people who have now been on this program – and when adhered to properly – ONLY normalised their weight.

The problem can be shown in a diagram. Assume your total calorie intake per day looks like this:

THE ANTI-CANDIDA DIET: A BASIS TO YOUR THERAPY

The shaded-in portion represents the amount of calories ingested via empty calorie foods (cakes, biscuits, white rice, fizzy drinks, and so on):

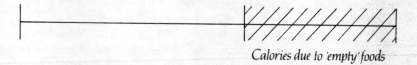

Calories due to 'empty' foods

These types of 'foods' provide energy, but no nourishment. The remainder of your dietary calorie intake (the unshaded area) hopefully is provided by more nourishing foods, such as fish, eggs, wholemeal pasta and much more.

When you start your anti-Candida diet the shaded area is immediately removed, decreasing your overall calorie intake and therefore creating weight loss unless you increase the quantity of allowable foods, the nourishing foods. If you are therefore overweight, your intake of such foods may have been adequate. This means that your intake of empty calorie foods was actually the source of your weight problem. Thus by cutting these out, your weight will normalise.

Other people will have had the majority of their total calorie intake from empty "foods". In this case, such items must be cut from their diet, but then it would also be necessary to increase the input of nourishing foods, to prevent drastic or sudden loss of weight.

Weight loss is an important issue. By adhering to the anti-Candida diet, which automatically removes all empty calorie substances, eating adequate amounts of balanced, nourishing foods you should *not* lose weight. This diet is restrictive in the *types* of foods you can eat, not in the *quantities* eaten.

Coffee and tea are problems for people who have Candida, not just because they contain caffeine, but rather, there is a fermentation process that the tea-leaves and coffee beans go through after picking, and hence the finished product contains traces of mould. This then exacerbates various symptoms of Candida. Over and above that of course, caffeine is hardly the thing to be pumping into an already ill and depleted body, thus further weakening the adrenals and liver. And that's not accounting for the negative effects it has on the nervous system.

As mentioned earlier, to give up coffee, tea, alcohol, cigarettes, sugar — all of a sudden and all at the same time — would require super-human effort. So let's look at a few hints on how to ease your way off these amazingly addictive substances. Many people refuse to believe this last statement . . . until they try to go "cold-turkey," when they can experience for themselves the withdrawal symptoms caused by giving these substances up too suddenly.

The elimination of coffee and tea is more easily achieved by the method of reduction. Obtain a small jar and fill it one quarter with a good quality decaffeinated coffee. Mix well and use till finished. Next time, mix half decaf and half real coffee together. When used up, then mix three-quarter decaff to one quarter real coffee, and finally of course you will be on pure decaff. The same applies to tea, which is also available in the decaffeinated form. This technique allows for a relatively smooth decrease in the amount of caffeine ingested, with a minimum of withdrawal symptoms.

To give up the decaff, simply reduce the quantity you drink, until you have cut out both the coffee and tea. The various coffee alternatives contain malt (a fermented type of sugar) and are not allowed in the anti-Candida diet. There are some exceptions available in most health food stores (see Appendix for further details). These could be substituted for the decaff in the reduction method.

Another issue that frequently arises is the dilemma of eating out, either at friends' places or in restaurants. The solutions are ridiculously easy: a) Eat a normal anti-Candida meal at home *before* you go to your host; b) Prepare your own meal and take it to your host; and c) Choose your restaurant carefully. Asian cuisine often uses MSG and much honey and sugar. Italian restaurants usually cook with a lot of cheese, sauces and commercially prepared tomato products, all of which could stir things up for you.

However, there are still many restaurants where you can get a grilled fish/meat/chicken dish or an omelette or a salad (no dressing). Such meals are adequate in nourishment and still allow you to go out with friends. Desserts are *all* a problem, unless you are able to tolerate fruit again, in which case you may have a freshly made fruit salad with no added sugar. Another frequent problem is that of people not making their own lunches and bringing these to work, and then finding little to eat if shopping around the "take-away" bars. Yet, there is a surprisingly nutritious lunch you CAN scratch together yourself, virtually anywhere a sandwich bar exists.

There is always a selection of various proteins such as chicken, egg or tinned fish. Then they also always have items such as lettuce, carrot, cucumber, onoions, capsium, tomato, avocado, if not more. These too are all totally safe to have.

So there you are in the middle of "fast-food land" and yet you can put together a lunch that will sustain you till you get home to your own supplies.

If things really look desperate, then ANYWHERE you go, you will always find a hamburger stall, or someone who sells fish and chips. Now, I would NEVER recommend these type of "foods" normally, but if the worst comes to the worst, you could simply throw away the hamburger bun and just eat the meat, or else peel off all the batter and only eat the fish.

Next, let's look more closely at exactly what you can and can't eat . . . and why."

3 THE ANTI-CANDIDA DIET: WHAT CAN I EAT?

It is important to have representatives from all the food groups in any diet that needs to be maintained for a length of time.

The first food group to look at are the proteins. There are two types: complete and incomplete. The first type contains all the essential amino acids our bodies require to reconstruct, heal and grow. These proteins are primarily found in animal sources. Incomplete proteins are lacking some of these essential amino acids and cannot provide all the building blocks the body needs, unless they are complemented. These proteins are mostly provided by plants.

Complementation is the process whereby two or more incomplete proteins are combined in the same meal, so that whatever amino acids one lacks the other provides. Hence, a meal is created supplying all the essential amino acids: a 'complete' protein meal.

This is basically vegetarianism, but it takes more dietetic knowledge, experience, time and commitment to provide complete and adequate protein nourishment over any length of time.

Meat, as a source of complete protein, is another controversial area that needs to be looked at. Some people are very surprised when I, a natural therapist, at times recommend meat. This is done for several reasons. Firstly, I have nothing against vegetarianism, as long as those who use this style of cooking and eating do so with full knowledge of the *science* of vegetarianism.

Very few people who work — especially working mothers — have an excess of that most precious of commodities, time. What happens to many vegetarians with busy lifestyles? They start to cut corners. Initially, the body can compensate, but eventually, especially when one is under stress, the complete or first-class protein requirements are not met, and the body starts to scavenge from its own organs and tissues.

The first loss is weight, but with time there is loss of organ and glandular tissue and hence function; ultimately, deep-seated ill-health sets in. This may not happen for six months, a year, possibly even several years. This depends on many factors, such as genetic constitution, stress levels, and 'break outs' from the pure vegetarian diet. The number of really sick vegetarians I have seen in my clinic over the years thoroughly appals me. When their situation is carefully looked into, the major problem is often the lack of adequate, complete protein over a long period of time, especially if associated with long-standing, heavy stress levels.

This is my main reason for pushing for complete sources of protein, those found in animal products. They include fish, chicken and eggs, and then last on the list the lighter meats such as lamb, veal or rabbit. I've also found that many people who have had severe Candida over a long period of time are often anaemic and greatly debilitated; they seem to feel better on at least some meat. Of course, if you have arthritis this could change the whole issue, yet even here there are levels to the situation that need to be carefully assessed.

Firstly, many cases of "arthritis" are in fact created by the Candida and as IT is taken care of, so the "arthritis" goes as well. Secondly, always listen to your body. If it tells you through a worsening of your symptoms, that meat does NOT suit you, then you MUST ignore me and listen to your body. The old saying of "one man's meat is another mans poison" couldn't be more appropriate here! For those living in the Sydney metropolitan area, a Biodynamic Meat Company does exist at 47a Spofforth St, Cremorne; 909-3383*

In this diet you can do quite well using vegetarian principles of combining vegetable sources of protein, but study this science of eating thoroughly. As far as chicken and eggs are concerned, it would be better if the free-range variety were procured.

Fresh fish is better, but again, is not always freely available. When you do have access to it, buy enough to last you perhaps several weeks, take it home and wrap them up into individual meal portions and freeze. This is far better — and still fresh enough and nourishing enough — than using tinned fish alone. The latter is okay in small amounts, but try to use only those tinned in plain oil not brine.

Although dairy foods are seen in our society as an important source of complete protein, it is not allowed on the Candida program, or only in minimal amounts. The processed dairy foods we use are especially prone to producing mucus in our bodies. This results in our systems becoming clogged and susceptible to malfunction, providing stagnant cesspools, as it were, in which Candida and other germs happily thrive.

It is a myth that if you don't eat dairy products, you'll end up with a calcium deficiency. As dairy products are so processed, most of the calcium is bound up in an unavailable form, and the mucus produced by dairy 'foods' prevents adequate absorption of nutrients through the bowel walls, because of the clogging effect of mucus. This includes absorption of calcium.

More than adequate amounts of calcium are obtained from a well-balanced diet which includes a wide range of green, leafy vegetables, nuts, seeds (especially sesame seed and Tahini, or sesame seed paste), as well as fish. You will

* Your local Natural Therapist's Association should be able to inform you about such possibilities in your area.

THE ANTI-CANDIDA DIET: WHAT CAN I EAT?

not become calcium deficient if you don't use dairy foods. Just make sure that the rest of your diet is balanced — as this anti-Candida diet is.

Milk substitutes are possible alternatives. There are many soy milks on the market, but the problem here is their palatability. Two of the best seem to be Bonsoy and its slightly more economical option, Vai Soy (see Appendix), both obtainable from health food stores.

Several other pleasant soy milks exist, such as "So-Good", but they are full of sugar and hence automatically out. Now we come to a sensitive and controversial point. The Bonsoy does contain malt (which is a fermented sugar) and theoretically should also be excluded from any anti-Candida diet. However, peoples' need for a dairy substitute are sometimes so high, that — with some trepidation! — I do allow them to at least TRY this milk alternative, but always on the understanding that if they do react to it, or if their overall progress isn't as fast as it should be, then this suspected item is immediately withdrawn. Another alternative is to make your own "nut-milk" according to the recipe given in Section III.

Although goat's milk on some levels is better tolerated by the human digestive system, it too cannot be used in this type of diet as it contains large amounts of lactose. The only form of dairy food that *is* allowed is butter. As it is the fat fraction of dairy produce, it contains no lactose and most people — even those allergic to the protein fraction — can handle butter.

Margarine is not an alternative. Never mind what they say in their advertising about how 'natural' it is, it is derived primarily from a chemically extracted oil, chemically hardened, chemically flavoured, chemically preserved, chemically emulsified . . . need I go on? Margarine is a chemical soup. Butter is a natural product, and you can nowadays get low- or no-salt butter.

Until now, we have dealt with the protein component of the anti-Candida diet. The next important food group to look at contains the carbohydrates or starches. These are provided mainly by the grains, the most important being rice, wheat, oats, barley, rye, millet, and buckwheat.

To obtain the full nourishing value of these sources of carbohydrate, they must be cooked and eaten in the *whole* grain form, that is, brown rice, wholemeal bread, wholemeal pasta. The white, processed grains, such as white rice, contain very little nourishment and plenty of calories.

If you were to plant a grain of brown rice and a grain of white rice, the white rice would rot and the brown rice would grow, simply because the brown rice is complete and contains all the nourishment necessary to produce life.

Another reason why wholegrains and wholegrain products are emphasised in the Candida diet is that besides providing more nourishment, the starch in

UNDERSTANDING CANDIDA

wholegrain foods is slow in breaking down in the digestive tract. There are no sudden floods of sugar (the breakdown product from starch) released into the system, which would only stimulate Candida growth.

Normal yeasted breads are definitely a problem for most people with Candida. Even though the bread has been baked and the yeast is dead, the substance from which the yeast is made, when ingested in foods such as bread, can still create a lot of suffering in your body. It is important to use bread that has not been yeasted, and this is available in most major cities.

Some of these breads use a very small amount of honey; this seems to cause no problems for the majority of people with Candida. If you are unfortunate enough to be so sensitive to honey that you do react, then refrain from using these breads.

It is better to buy several loaves at a time, especially if they are hard for you to obtain, and then slice and freeze them. You will be less likely to run out of yeast-free bread and less tempted to resort to 'normal' bread.

There are also wholemeal crumpets which contain baking soda instead of yeast. These seem safe for most people with Candida and can be eaten for a change and a treat. Other than these sources of breads, there are several recipes given later in this book for bread/damper/scones/pancakes and flapjacks.

Several different types of biscuits such as rice cakes and Ryvitas exist which contain no yeast. Always read the labels for yeast or sugar content. Don't be fooled by the words 'no sugar added'. Sugar in this instance legally means sucrose which is only one of many different forms of sugar. When they have this on the label they mean that this product contains no sucrose, but it may be laden with glucose, fructose, maltose, hexose or dextrose: *all* these are sugars too! Such products must not be eaten.

Starches are also obtained from various vegetables, especially the root vegetables such as potatoes, carrots, parsnips, turnips, beetroot, and pumpkin. If you are allergic to all grains, you can still get your starch requirements from these foods. When such items are eaten in moderate amounts, as part of an overall meal, they present no problems in this diet. However, if you do as some of my clients did, and have whole platefuls of mashed potato, pumpkin or carrot, then you are bound to experience problems!!

Perhaps one to be a little wary of is white potato. Research evidence from St Vincent's Hospital in Sydney, where they tested white potato prepared in various ways to see how it affected the blood sugar levels of diabetics, concluded that the starch in white potato broke down to sugar units in the body so rapidly that the effect on the blood sugar levels was virtually the same as taking a tablespoon of sugar or honey. Mashed potato was the worst culprit and fried chips the least,

THE ANTI-CANDIDA DIET: WHAT CAN I EAT?

due to the amount of fat in the chips greatly slowing down the rate at which the body was able to digest it. (No, this does *not* justify eating fried chips!)

It is best to leave white potato out of the diet altogether for about the same time that fruits are initially forbidden (four to eight weeks). You could consider experimenting with dry-baked potatoes as a small addition to the diet. Here the potato is simply placed in a hot oven for about two hours or so, till cooked. Strangely enough, sweet potato doesn't seem to cause as many problems as white potato in regard to increasing sugar levels and therefore feeding Candida, so it is seen on the same level as pumpkin, carrot or other such vegetables, as a *portion* of a serve in an overall meal. Let your body tell you if this is so or not.

The next food group to consider includes the vegetables and fruits. These are both important as they provide substantial nourishment in the form of vitamins, minerals, starches and even small amounts of protein. Fruits are not allowed in the initial weeks of Candida therapy, simply because they are so high in sugar and will exacerbate Candida growth at a time when we are especially trying to stifle such activity by the fungus. Virtually all vegetables are allowed, with two exceptions: sweet corn on the cob and as discussed, white potato. Other than these two, freedom of choice is yours, including such items as avocado and tomato. All vegetables must be fresh, without mouldy patches. Certain foods such as zucchini, pumpkin and tomato are prone to mould and should be carefully inspected before cooking. All vegetables should be eaten either lightly steamed or raw.

Don't take the raw food fad too far. There are some foods, the root vegetables particularly, that need to be cooked. If we were cows it would be a different matter. They have several stomachs, some of which act like fermentation vats or stoves. We have only one stomach and it certainly isn't able to act like a stove. That piece of equipment is found in the kitchen, and should be used!

Although small amounts of juice from lemons or limes can be used in cooking from the very beginning of the diet, certain fruits such as the various berries should be avoided for most of the period of treatment. They may be resumed once the system has had a chance to stabilise and heal. These fruits are particularly susceptible to mould and are too much of a risk. Other fruits such as rockmelon and papaw are also prone to mould and, although they are allowed after the initial four to eight weeks, eat with great care. Check them thoroughly for any mouldy spots before eating.

This is where some diets for Candida therapy go to extremes. Anything and everything that may have mould in or on it is banned. This leaves very little that can be totally guaranteed to be yeast or mould free. The very air that you breathe contains moulds and yeasts. Does this mean you should wear a mask

UNDERSTANDING CANDIDA

twenty-fours hours a day? A sense of balance needs to be maintained with a pinch of commonsense to provide good results in therapy, and to make life at least livable!

Nuts and seeds are a most valuable and important source of protein and there is no reason to neglect these in a Candida program. Ensure that they are as fresh as possble by going to stores that have a good reputation for quality goods, and to stores that are busy (stock is more likely to be 'turned over' quickly). The nuts are less likely to have been sitting on the shelves for years, growing mouldy, perhaps rancid.

Nuts and seeds make an ideal snack between meals and for this reason pose a potential problem. If you have Candida, you may be allergic to some foods. An allergy is more likely if you eat the same food day in, day out.

Nuts could easily fall into this category. If you eat nuts on a daily basis, rotate the varieties every few days. It makes the nuts less boring to eat, and the risk of an allergy reaction is greatly reduced.

Nuts and seeds can be a valuable addition to various recipes and have been included in some in this book (there is always room for further experimentation). Various nut 'butters' are now available from health food stores, such as cashew butter and hazelnut butter. These are safe and delicious as spreads or toppings.

The nuts to be careful of are pistachio and peanuts, as they could be contaminated by mould. As your health improves, you may reintroduce peanuts, freshly roasted in the shell or as peanut butter.

The final food group are the oils. Chemically extracted oils, routinely bought in grocery stores, may present a health hazard. It is far better to buy cold-pressed oils from your health food store. These are more expensive, but are purer, more nutritious and bear no traces of poisonous chemicals left behind during processing. There are many types of cold-pressed oils available, but two that are especially therapeutic for anyone with a Candida problem are safflower and olive oil. Safflower oil contains traces of the essential fatty acids normally found in other products such as Evening Primrose Oil (very expensive!). Olive oil has the ability to keep Candida in the non-pathogenic yeast form, in our gut.

Such oils are needed in any diet for optimum health, and should be included in food preparation, either as a salad dressing, in stir-frying or simply taken in a teaspoon (1 to 6 teaspoons a day).

THE ANTI-CANDIDA DIET: WHAT CAN I EAT?

A SUMMARY

PROTEINS
- All fish, fowl, eggs, meat (lighter types).
- All vegetarian protein combinations.
- Dairy products are specifically excluded (except for small quantities of cottage cheese, with care).

CARBOHYDRATES (starches)
- All grains and wholegrain products, including bread in the yeast-free form (read the label).
- Certain vegetables.

FRUITS AND VEGETABLES
- All vegetables are allowed (except for sweet corn and white potato in the early stages of treatment).
- All fruit, including fruit juice and carrot juice (lemon/lime juice in small quantities is allowed) are definitely *out* for the first 4 to 8 weeks. Slowly reintroduce them as tolerated.

FATS, OILS
- Butter is fine. No margarine.
- Cold-pressed oils are good, especially safflower and olive oil.

This selection is balanced and any diet of these items will provide a solid basis to long-term health.

4 THE ANTI-CANDIDA DIET: WHAT CAN'T I EAT?

Having looked at all the permissible foods, and realising that virtually all the basic foods we normally eat are still 'in', what is 'out'? Many of the items that are not allowed are those 'nice' extras we have grown so used to, to the point of accepting them as normal, rather than as a luxury aspect to our diets.

Candida thrives on sugars, and a person who is filled with Candida-produced toxins reacts strongly to anything yeasty or mouldy. Anything that contains moderate to high levels of sugar (cakes, sweets, biscuits, fizzy drinks, chocolates as well as fruit, fruit juice, carrot juice and honey) is definitely out. This area also includes such 'foods' as white bread, white pasta (even the green pasta, as it is nothing but white pasta with added green colouring) and refined grains and their flours.

Processed foods, whether tinned or packaged, are largely not allowed as they usually contain sugars and yeast or MSG (derived from yeast), as well as artificial flavourings, preservatives, emulsifiers, and so on. Dried fruits are especially out as they are not only concentrated in sugar, but also frequently contain mould.

Next on the list of 'out' items is anything made by or made from yeasts or moulds. A person with Candida is highly sensitive to anything yeasty and will react — often very dramatically — to anything ingested that is of a yeasty nature. Items such as Vegemite, Promite, soy sauce, pure yeast, mushrooms (a fungus), beer, wine, spirits and vinegars are not allowed. Cheeses become mouldy, if not actively filled with mould (for example, camembert, brie or blue vein). As a dairy item they are a double no-no!

Breads containing yeasts are out. Anything containing citric acid is out, as it is derived from yeast. Malted products, such as breakfast cereals, alternative 'coffees', Horlicks, Milo, are out, as they contain maltose (a sugar).

Coffees and teas are out. All processed meats and smoked meats, including processed sandwich meats, are out. Condiments such as mustards, pickles and mayonnaise are out as they usually contain vinegar, a fermented product.

Although a staple Western food (dairy produce) is virtually eliminated from the diet, it still leaves an ample choice of foods to be eaten. The problems begin if you are someone who has done most of their eating in restaurants or from take-aways. These types of food are invariably filled or laced with many forbidden items. Foods prepared as Nature provided them are nourishing and strengthening and need not be boring.

Although various condiments are out, all the culinary herbs and spices are definitely in. You can use fresh supplies of such products with ingenuity and abandon to produce very tasty meals. These herbs can be in either the green form (straight from your herb garden), or dried (these need to be of excellent quality to avoid mould).

Once having cooked or prepared the food, there is an art to eating it properly. Many of us in our high-speed society are always on the go, even when we're eating. This does untold harm to our digestive systems, especially if it becomes a regular way of eating: it is not only when physically active that it is harmful to eat, but also when stressed.

Our nervous system is divided into two main branches, the sympathetic and the parasympathetic. The first is involved in preparing us for trouble (the system that switches on for the fight or flight response). This is where you get a rush of adrenalin, your heart beats faster, your blood pressure goes up and all your daily 'household' chores within your body — such as maintenance and repair, *as well as digestion* — are stopped. It is only when the parasympathetic nervous system is active (a sedate, relaxed state of being), that we are able to adequately digest and absorb our food, allowing all our body functions to be nourished and repaired.

Within the body, only one system can be operative at any one time. As we live in such a hectic, stressed environment, either at home or at work, the sympathetic nervous system is usually operating. In this mode, we *cannot* adequately digest our food. The food stagnates in our bowels or stomachs, eventually fermenting and producing massive amounts of toxic byproducts which are absorbed into our bodies. It is very important to maximise our parasympathetic nervous system function before we sit down to eat. Eating 'on the hoof' or while stressed cancels this possibility. Despite our deadlines and the harried lifestyles we must *make* time to eat in as peaceful a setting and manner as possible, if we want to maintain our health.

A very natural, easy way to increase your digestive powers is by ensuring that fresh, live seed sprouts are eaten with each meal. These not only contain concentrated amounts of vitamins, minerals, proteins and starches, but also many valuable enzymes that help your stomach to digest food. Virtually every greengrocer sells alfalfa or mung bean sprouts nowadays. There is also a very simple way of growing these at home. All you need is a wide-necked glass jar, some nylon mosquito mesh to place over the top of the jar, a strong elastic band to hold it in place, your selection of seeds to be sprouted, such as alfalfa, mung, lentil, mustard, fenugreek or many others, a warm spot to keep the jar in and only a few minutes a day to quickly rinse and drain the growing sprouts. Place from one to three tablespoons of seed into a one-litre glass jar. Secure the mesh with the elastic band over the mouth of the jar. Pour water into the jar, through

THE ANTI-CANDIDA DIET: WHAT CAN'T I EAT?

the mesh. Stand for 12 hours or so, and drain by inverting the jar (the mesh will keep the seed inside). Rinse and drain the seed several times until the run-off water is clear. Drain for about one minute and then place the jar on its side in a warm, light spot, out of direct sunlight. Rinse and drain the bottle every day, until the seed has sprouted enough (usually after seven to ten days). Give the sprouts a final, thorough rinse and then drain for five minutes. Remove the sprouts from the jar and place in a plastic bag, squeezing out all the air. Seal and store in the fridge. Add a handful of sprouts to as many meals as you can. Don't let the sprouts go slimy or mouldy, as this will lead to Candida problems. If the process has been done correctly and the sprouts have been stored for only five to six days at a time, no complications should arise.

What do we do with left-over food: throw it away or store it? Many therapists will say 'throw it away' as storing food results in mould. If the food has been carefully produced from clean sources and has not been left uncovered, then there is no reason why such food can't be safely frozen for some months, or stored in the fridge for at least one to two days. After that, some mould will start to form.

The most urgent question clients need to have answered is when can they start fruit again? There is no standard answer to this as it depends on how you have progressed under the anti-Candida program. In most cases, if people have made a very concerted effort and have adhered to the diet and the medications, I find that their symptoms have improved so much by the fourth, fifth or sixth week that it is feasible to very cautiously reintroduce small amounts of fruit (such as a tiny kiwi fruit, a quarter of an apple or pear, a small slice of papaw, or any other fruit that is not too sweet). Do this for about a week and see how you feel. If you continue to improve without the return of the various aches and other symptoms you may carefully increase your fruit intake by an extra portion every week. It is important to make only a small increase per day for an entire week before taking more, as sometimes it can take several days before you notice a decline in your overall status.

To summarise: All sugary foods and drinks (including sugar of natural sources) are out. All yeasty, fermented, fungus items are out. They will directly or indirectly make your Candida symptoms worse. Other than dairy foods, everything that is removed from your diet is a non-essential luxury item.

You are left with more than enough of all the various food groups, to provide you with a very adequate, balanced nourishment. Yeast-free/sugar-free cooking need not be bland nor boring. Use the recipes provided and embellish them if you wish, with whatever culinary herbs and spices that are available. Sprouted seeds are an easy-to-prepare and valuable addition to your diet. Food left-overs can be

UNDERSTANDING CANDIDA

safely stored in the freezer for months, or in the fridge for several days; always package properly. Finally, remember that stress and eating are not compatible bedmates.

SECTION III

Recipes . . . and Further Hints

1 INFORMATION ON THE 14-DAY ROTATION DIET

In any text like this only a general guideline can be given, because each person's needs will be different. Primarily, only the safest recipes have been chosen for the 14-day rotation program, suitable for anyone who is suffering from Candida.

For people who are beyond the initial stages of Candida therapy, and whose symptoms have settled down, they need not adhere to all restrictions; they may 'open up' their diet to the extent they feel is safe.

For most people it may be best to start this program on a Saturday, simply because it may be easier to complete the first week's shopping from the list provided. Also, the weekend may be used to organise and precook some of your lunches for the coming week.

Yeast-free bread, fish, chicken or meat may easily be frozen, if needed. Package individually for each meal and organise the freezer for easy access to each day's requirements.

To maximise the benefits of this section it is advisable to have first read the book thus far to understand exactly why you need to make changes to your diet. Next, thoroughly read through the recipes for the 14 days to see where there may be problems for you.

Always plan ahead: you will be less likely to be caught short or unprepared, minimising the chances of you going off the diet. Once you are familiar with the program, check the program summary (see Appendix), which is detachable and should be taken from the book and stuck somewhere in your kitchen where it will be easy to refer to at a glance.

The recipe section contains a series of reminders which will prompt you to take certain items from the freezer, or prepare certain foods in advance. Again, this minimises the chances of going off the diet.

Each recipe is planned for two people, unless otherwise stated. To serve meals for more, simply multiply the ingredients by the desired number.

Below is a list of definitions of concepts and words used in the recipe section.

- 'loaf' = a yeast-free bread.
- 'milk' = any brand of soy milk, preferably without malt/sugars, or 'nut' milk (see Index).
- 'oil' = any cold-pressed vegetable oil. Especially good is a 1:1 blend of safflower and olive oils. (Note: *saf*flower and *sun*flower are not the same.)
- 'tomato paste' = homemade paste using tomatoes (see Index).

- 'salt' = any rock salt, especially a good, herbally flavoured salt.
- 'spices' = any of the normal household spices, such as cinnamon, nutmeg, cloves, allspice, fennel, anise, ground ginger, mixed spice.
- 'spreads' = a specially formulated spread or topping for such things as sandwiches, pancakes and flapjacks. Can be used as a sauce in a recipe (see Index).
- 'sprouts' = sprouted seeds, not brussels sprouts.

The measurement of quantity for the herbs and spices in any recipe depends very much on your tastes. Some people like their foods very spicy; others can handle nothing but the very mildest of dishes. Experiment and see what your needs are. In a few cases, exact amounts have been advised.

Breakfast
Some people can't stomach a full breakfast first thing in the morning! There are several options available. Firstly, instead of breakfast, have a cup of C-Herb Tea. The herbs in the tea improve the appetite; perhaps before too long you will be able to cope with a good breakfast.

Secondly, select at least two to three different breakfast menus from this book; choose the ones you would most likely be able to manage, and then rotate these. The more you find to rotate, the better it will be.

Most people who skip breakfast find themselves hungry at work. What will you find to eat at or near work? Not much: coffee, sticky buns, pies, biscuits, takeaways... You could prepare a take-from-home breakfast, such as sandwiches, wholemeal scones or muesli or perhaps some protein in the form of a boiled egg, chicken leg or nuts.

Breakfast is an important meal which should not be skipped. When you initially look at some of the breakfast recipes, it would be very easy to react with "these would take too long!" or "I haven't got the time for this first thing in the morning!" And then it would be all too enticing to just have that bowl of muesli by itself. On one level that is of course very nutritious and Okay. However, this 14-day recipe program has been planned to provide a wide range of rotatable foods, minimising the risk of creating allergies. Many of the breakfasts can be made at a convenient time and then reheated. An example would be the fish. This could be very easily prepared the night before. First thing in the morning, light the oven and put in your breakfast. Then have your shower and get dressed. By this time your meal should be ready. Organise yourself... that will be the key to your success!

INFORMATION ON THE 14-DAY ROTATION DIET

Lunch
Lunches, too, need some effort in preparation and organisation. For some who have no heating facilities at work, the type of lunches as discussed here may be unworkable. In that case, select a number of recipes that are easy and practical for you to have as lunches, and rotate these around.

Remember that if the worst comes to the worst any sandwich bar will offer something nourishing, in accordance with the Candida regime.

For those who want a quickie salad, place a slice of cucumber, tomato, carrot, lettuce and capsicum in a small container, with a dollop of sprouts on top. That type of salad takes no time at all, and is full of goodness.

As there is a heavy emphasis on including adequate quantities of fresh, raw greens in the Candida diet, the lunches are structured to include a salad. Where you see salad in the menu, look at the choices provided later in the book (see Index). Choose one for that day. These few suggestions are not the be-all and end-all of your salad choices: by all means go ahead and *experiment*! Devise variations using combinations of your favourite foods and your favourite vegetables, as they come into season. Remember to follow the Candida guidelines as outlined earlier in this book, to avoid possible food-allergy reactions.

Dinner
The recipes given for dinnertime meals are aimed at providing simple, easy-to-prepare, nutritious food. The aim is to provide a balance of protein, complex carbohydrate, vegetables and oil. For people *starting* the Candida diet, the simple answer to the whole issue of desserts is... NO! Every recipe you might choose, has fruit or some source of sweetness in it and therefore is automatically out.

Later, as your condition stabilises and as your practitioner advises, fruit may be added after meals as a dessert. For those initial weeks without fruit, a piece of capsicum or a small piece of raw carrot may be eaten: this helps to satisfy some sweet cravings.

Vegetables can be either lightly steamed or cut up finely and stir fried in some oil. You may choose a salad instead of steamed vegetables. If there are ingredients in these dinner recipes that you know you can't tolerate or you don't like to eat, substitute something else that is within the boundaries of the Candida diet. For instance, these recipes use a lot of onions and garlic, intentionally, for their medicinal effect. However, if you find the quantity of garlic is too much for you, reduce the amount or leave it out.

The roasts have been organised for the weekends, simply because you may then have more time to spend in the kitchen. You can, of course, move the menus around to better suit your schedule.

Soups can always be served for an easy entree. Large quantities can be made at a time and frozen in special storage containers, until needed. There is no need to defrost: remove from the freezer and heat in a pan. Bring to the boil for one to two minutes before serving.

2 SHOPPING LIST FOR WEEK ONE

It's time to buy your first week's worth of 'goodies'. For those not used to eating or cooking at home, such staple items as herbs, spices, tahini and nut butters may not be stocked on your shelves. So, this first shopping list will be a little longer than next week's. Cross out the items you know you already have. To make it easier, the lists have been divided into groups such as grocer, butcher and health food store.

You may prefer to buy the vegetables daily, or all at once. It would be better to buy the vegetables daily or every few days, as you are less likely to encounter mould problems. However, this should not occur if the vegetables are properly cleaned and stored. Some books on Candida suggest that the vegetables be washed in water with bleach to kill mould spores. Do *not* follow this type of advice! Bleach is a poison, no matter how diluted. You already get more than enough chlorine from your tap water! It would be difficult to remove all of this bleach, even with repeated rinsing. Wetting vegetables, even if you try to dry them afterwards, will in itself result in excessive moisture during storage, *enhancing* further mould growth.

As you look through the recipes, you'll see that in several cases you are given a choice; for example, vegetables or salad, soup or stew. Your shopping lists will depend very much on what you choose to have.

As everyone's idea of what constitutes a serving is somewhat different, these shopping lists — in some areas such as vegetables — may not quite fit your needs. By making adjustments to these lists, future shopping should be accurate and trouble-free.

SHOPPING LIST: WEEK ONE

GROCER
- Mixed herbs
- Plain chilli or a blend of chilli with other herbs/spices
- Cinnamon
- Nutmeg
- Oregano
- Rosemary
- Curry powder
- Basil
- Dry mustard powder
- Marjoram

- Paprika
- Coriander
- Dill
- Bay leaves
- Mixed spice
- Turmeric
- Cardamom
- 2×185g tins tuna/salmon (preferably in brine or oil)
- 1×250g tin tuna/salmon
- 250g cottage cheese
- Baking powder
- 1½ dozen eggs (preferably free range)
- Kebab sticks
- 1 to 2 tins sardines (for sandwiches)

BUTCHER
- 4 chicken drumsticks
- 1 leg of lamb
- 200g lamb's fry (liver)
- 750g chicken mince
- 250g diced veal
- 2 large chicken breast fillets
- 1 medium chicken, for soup (preferably free range)
- 1kg veal mince

FISH
- 250g fish fillets (boneless)

HEALTH FOOD STORE
- 2 to 3 yeast-free bread loaves
- 1kg sunflower seeds
- 500g sesame seeds
- 500g nuts of your choice, or mixed
- 1 pkt wholemeal pasta
- 1 litre oil (cold pressed)
- Rock salt (preferably flavoured with herbal extracts)
- 1 large jar tahini
- 1kg lentils
- 1 jar hazelnut butter

SHOPPING LIST FOR WEEK 1

- 1 jar cashew butter
- 1 small pkt tofu
- 1 pkt yeast and sugar-free biscuits
- 1 to 2 pkts ricecakes
- 500g chick peas
- soy milk (with no sugar or yeast/malt)
- 500g almonds (if you wish to make nut milk)
- 1¼kg rolled oats
- 1 container pure protein powder (no sugars or starches)
- 500g flaxseed
- 500g pipetas
- 250g bran
- 250g wheat germ
- 250g hulled millet
- 2kg wholemeal, self-raising flour
- 500g gluten flour
- 500g buckwheat flour
- 500g cornmeal
- 1 to 2 vanilla beans
- 500g pure carob powder
- 500g buckwheat
- 1 pkt wholemeal pastry
- 1kg brown rice

GREENGROCER
- 3 medium pieces sweet potato
- 1 small bunch beetroot
- 1 large piece pumpkin
- 4 parsnips
- 2 lettuce
- 1 bunch radish
- 2 cucumbers
- 3kg tomato (2kg for the tomato paste)
- 6 medium zucchini
- 1 whole celery
- 4 capsicums
- 2 containers sprouts
- 2 bunches chives
- ½ cabbage

- 1kg carrots
- 1 large bunch parsley
- 2kg onions
- 1 bunch fresh basil (if available)
- 10 lemons
- 3 avocado
- 2 cloves garlic
- 100g ginger
- 500g beans
- ½ cauliflower
- 250g brussels sprouts
- Fresh rosemary
- Fresh mint
- 1 leek
- 1 bunch silverbeet
- 1 large eggplant
- 100g peas
- 1 head broccholi
- Anything else that you may like to add

3 MENU FOR WEEK ONE: BREAKFAST, LUNCH, DINNER

BREAKFAST WEEK 1 DAY 1
- Chicken drumsticks
- Steamed vegetables
- C-Herb Tea

1 TO 4 CHICKEN DRUMSTICKS

A SELECTION OF VEGETABLES, FOR EXAMPLE, SPRING BEANS, BRUSSELS SPROUTS, BROCCOLI, CAULIFLOWER, ZUCCHINI, CARROT, PUMPKIN AND SWEET POTATO (the latter two in small portions only)

HERBS/SPICES

Strip the skin from the drumsticks. Sprinkle with salt, herbs and spices. Wrap in foil or place in a casserole dish. Cook in the oven at 200°C for 20 to 25 minutes.

Wash or peel vegetables and place in a steamer. Steam for 5 to 10 minutes (the time will depend on the vegetables used). Do not overcook the vegetables; they should still be crisp. Serve with the drumsticks. Tahini, sauces or spreads may be added for flavour. Herbs or spices may also be sprinkled over the meal.

Drink 1 cup of C-Herb Tea, preferably before the meal.

LUNCH WEEK 1 DAY 1
- Tuna
- Salad
- Loaf
- C-Herb Tea

1 × 185g TIN TUNA (preferably in brine)

SALAD (see Index)

BUTTERED SLICES OF LOAF

Choose the salad you would like today. Prepare. Drain and remove tuna from tin. Place both tuna and salad in a lunch box. Butter required number of slices of loaf and pack separately. Heat C-Herb Tea in the morning and take to work in a thermos. Drink one cup before lunch (it stimulates the gastric juices) or at morning or afternoon teatime.

Serves one.

DINNER WEEK 1 DAY 1
- Roast lamb and vegetables
- Steamed broccoli or salad
- C-Herb Tea

1 LEG OF LAMB (lean as possible)

2 SMALL PIECES EACH OF SWEET POTATO, BEETROOT, PUMPKIN AND PARSNIP

4 TO 5 SMALL CLOVES OF GARLIC

3 TO 4 SPRIGS OF FRESH ROSEMARY

OIL

MASTERFOODS MEXICAN STYLE CHILLI (or similar chilli mixture)

SALT/PEPPER (optional)

MIXED HERBS

2 SERVINGS OF BROCCOLI

3 HEAPED TABLESPOONS FRESH MINT

80g BUTTER

1 TABLESPOON LEMON JUICE

Peel the cloves of garlic and insert them into stab holes in the lamb. Insert sprigs of rosemary into the stab holes. Seal the open end of the leg by searing it on the hot, oiled surface of a frypan. Sprinkle the leg with salt, pepper, chilli and mixed herbs. Wrap the leg in foil and place on a baking tray. Prepare the root vegetables and baste them in oil. Also place on the baking tray. Put into the oven at 180°C for 1½ hours. Then unwrap the lamb from the foil and return to the oven.

While the lamb is cooking, prepare the mint butter by chopping the fresh mint very finely. Allow the butter to soften before vigorously mixing in the mint, lemon juice, salt and pepper with a fork. Put in the refrigerator to harden the butter before serving with the roast lamb. Steam the broccoli and serve with the roast lamb and vegetables.

Drink 1 cup of C-Herb Tea, preferably before the meal.

Left-over lamb can be used in sandwiches.

HINT: Remove portion of frozen stew/soup for tomorrow's lunch, *or* decide to make now. Will also need it for breakfast on Day 6.

MENU FOR WEEK I: BREAKFAST, LUNCH, DINNER

BREAKFAST WEEK 1 DAY 2
- Lamb's fry and onions with tomato and sprouts
- Loaf or wholemeal scones
- C-Herb Tea

1 SMALL ONION
OIL
LAMB'S FRY (170g)
1 SMALL TOMATO
SPROUTS
LOAF OR WHOLEMEAL SCONES (see Index)

It is a good idea to have a supply of frozen wholemeal scones. Take the required number from the freezer, wrap them in foil and place in the oven at 220°C for 15 minutes or so.

While they're warming, peel and chop the onion. Saute in oil until brown. Wash the tomato and slice in half. Place in frypan with the onions. Slice the liver into thin strips about 2cm thick and add to the other ingredients in the pan. Cook each side of liver for about 5 minutes.

Serve with the hot buttered scones, and a small handful of sprouts.
Drink 1 cup of C-Herb Tea, preferably before the meal.
Serves one.

> HINT: Soak the lentils for tonight's dahl.

LUNCH WEEK 1 DAY 2
- Soup/stew
- Loaf
- Sprouts
- C-Herb Tea

ONE PORTION OF SOUP OR STEW

BUTTERED SLICES OF LOAF WITH ANY SPREAD (see Index)

SPROUTS

THERMOS

Butter and spread the loaf either in the morning or the evening before.

If you do not have facilities for heating your soup or stew at work, buy a wide-necked Thermos and quickly heat the soup/stew before you leave home. To speed up the process in the morning, remove the frozen portion of soup or stew the night before to allow it to thaw out overnight.

Sprinkle the sprouts on to the soup/stew, or have as a sidedish with the loaf.
Drink 1 cup of C-Herb Tea, preferably before the meal.

MENU FOR WEEK I: BREAKFAST, LUNCH, DINNER

DINNER WEEK 1 DAY 2
- Dahl pancake roll
- Steamed vegetables or salad
- C-Herb Tea

1 CUP LENTILS
3 BAY LEAVES
1 LEEK OR 1 MEDIUM ONION
OIL
3cm GINGER ROOT
2 TABLESPOONS CHOPPED PARSLEY
2 CLOVES GARLIC
TURMERIC/CARDAMOM/CINNAMON/PAPRIKA
SALT/PEPPER (optional)
MASTERFOODS MEXICAN STYLE CHILLI (or similar)
ROSEMARY/OREGANO/MARJORAM
¾ CUP TOMATO PASTE
1 TEASPOON TAHINI
CHOICE OF VEGETABLES FOR STEAMING OR FOR A SALAD

Presoak the lentils or do a 'quick soak' (see Index). Rinse well. Add the bay leaves and simmer for 25 minutes or until cooked. Meanwhile, chop the leek and saute until brown or soft. Add the remaining ingredients and mix well. Strain the cooked lentils, mash and mix with the other ingredients. Set aside. Make the pancakes. Spread the pancakes with the dahl mix and roll up. Wrap in foil or, preferably, place in a casserole dish. Heat in an oven at 200°C for 15 to 20 minutes. Serve with the vegetables or salad. Pour Ginger Sauce (see Index) over the top of the pancake roll.

> *HINT:* Make the quiche now for tomorrow's lunch, if you're working. Soak the buckwheat now for tomorrow's breakfast.

BREAKFAST WEEK 1 DAY 3
- Buckwheat and rolled oats porridge
- Mixed nuts
- C-Herb Tea

40g ROLLED OATS (or any rolled/'flaked' grain)
20g BUCKWHEAT
450ml WATER, OR MILK
KNOB OF BUTTER OR 1 TO 2 TEASPOONS OIL
CINNAMON/NUTMEG
1 TEASPOON ROASTED SESAME SEEDS
DESIRED AMOUNT OF MIXED NUTS

Soak the buckwheat overnight in the 450ml of water or milk. Bring to the boil, add the rolled oats, then simmer very slowly for 5 to 10 minutes. Before serving, add cinnamon or nutmeg and mix in well. Finally add the butter or oil and sprinkle with the roasted sesame seeds. These can be freshly roasted by placing in a heavy, unoiled frypan. Heat. Stir the sesame seeds until they go golden brown. It is best to prepare only as many as you would use in a week of cooking.

Drink 1 cup of C-Herb Tea, preferably before the meal.
Serves one.

> **HINT:** Remove the fish from freezer for tonight's casserole.

LUNCH WEEK 1 DAY 3
- Quiche
- Salad
- C-Herb Tea

WHOLEMEAL PASTRY
2 SMALL ONIONS
1 CLOVE GARLIC
80g CAPSICUM
1 SMALL TOMATO
OIL
1 TABLESPOON TOMATO PASTE
6 EGGS

MENU FOR WEEK I: BREAKFAST, LUNCH, DINNER

60g TOFU
SALT/PEPPER (optional)
HERBS (Mixed herbs/rosemary/parsley)
PAPRIKA
MILK
PINCH MUSTARD POWDER
BUTTER
SESAME SEEDS

Chop one onion, saute in oil until brown. Add chopped garlic. Meanwhile, place the pastry in a greased quiche tin and blind-bake* for 15 minutes. A number of smaller quiches can be made by using a cupcake baking tray.

Finely dice the capsicum and tomato and add to the onions and garlic. Add the eggs, tomato paste, tofu, a dash of milk and the herbs and spices together and mix briefly in a blender.

Once the pastry has been blind-baked, remove the foil, place the sauteed ingredients on the bottom of the pastry and pour the blended egg mix over this. Put a few slices of tomato on top. Spread some finely chopped onion over this and finish off with a sprinkle of sesame seeds. Place in oven at 180°C for 30 to 40 minutes.

Serve hot or cold with salad.

Drink 1 cup of C-Herb Tea, preferably before the meal.

Spare quiche makes a good snack for later. Store in the fridge.

*Blind-baking: line the quiche tin with the pastry. Over this place some foil and then fill with something to keep the pastry in place. After 15 minutes or so, take from the oven. Remove the filling and the foil and continue with the recipe.

UNDERSTANDING CANDIDA

DINNER WEEK 1 DAY 3
- Fish casserole
- Wholemeal noodles
- Steamed vegetables
- C-Herb Tea

1 SMALL ONION
OIL
2 HEAPED TABLESPOONS WHOLEMEAL FLOUR
SALT/PEPPER (optional)
250g FISH FILLETS (boneless)
1 SMALL CUCUMBER
½ LEMON
1 MEDIUM TOMATO
½ CUP WHOLEMEAL NOODLES
¾ CUP TOMATO PASTE
MASTERFOODS MEXICAN STYLE CHILLI/CURRY POWDER/PINCH OF DILL
CHOICE OF VEGETABLES FOR STEAMING, OR A SALAD

Chop onion and saute in oil until brown. Add flour, spices and herbs together in a plastic bag. Cut up the fish into small pieces and toss in the seasoned flour in the bag. Add fish and remaining flour to onions and stir fry for 5 minutes. Add extra oil if necessary.

Meanwhile, cut the cucumber in lengths. Remove the seed and chop into chunks. Place fish into casserole dish. Add chopped cucumber and tomato pieces. Add the juice from the lemon and the tomato paste. Cover and place in oven at 200°C for 45 minutes.

Meanwhile, prepare the pasta by boiling it in water for about 10 to 20 minutes (test occasionally until cooked).

Serve the fish over the pasta, with the steamed vegetables or salad.

Drink 1 cup of C-Herb Tea, preferably before the meal.

MENU FOR WEEK I: BREAKFAST, LUNCH, DINNER

BREAKFAST WEEK 1 DAY 4
- Scrambled eggs
- Loaf toast
- C-Herb Tea

2 EGGS
1 TABLESPOON MILK
1 TABLESPOON OIL
1 SMALL ONION OR 1 CLOVE OF GARLIC
CHIVES
HERBS/SPICES
DESIRED NUMBER OF SLICES OF LOAF
SPROUTS

Finely chop up the onion/garlic. Saute in oil until brown. Add eggs, milk and herbs/spices together and mix gently. Pour this over the browned onions/garlic and slowly stir until cooked. Meanwhile, toast the loaf. Serve the scrambled eggs on the hot toast. Sprinkle chopped chives over the top and add some sprouts as a sidedish.

Preferably have the C-Herb Tea before the meal.
Serves one.

HINT: Remove mince from freezer for tonight's shepherd's pie and tomorrow's meat balls.

85

LUNCH WEEK 1 DAY 4
- Mixed nuts and seeds
- Salad
- Wholemeal scones
- C-Herb Tea

MIXED NUTS AND SEEDS

SALAD

WHOLEMEAL SCONES (from freezer)

THERMOS OF C-HERB TEA

Measure out the desired amount of mixed nuts. Prepare the salad. Remove wholemeal scones from the freezer. Wrap in foil and reheat in oven at 220°C, for about 15 minutes.

Serve the nuts and seeds, salad and scones together.

Preferably have the C-Herb Tea before the meal.

MENU FOR WEEK 1: BREAKFAST, LUNCH, DINNER

DINNER WEEK 1 DAY 4
- Shepherd's pie
- Steamed vegetables or salad
- C-Herb Tea

500g MINCE (CHICKEN OR VEAL)
1 SMALL ONION
3 CLOVES OF GARLIC (optional)
1 CUP EACH OF CHOPPED OR DICED SWEET POTATO, PUMPKIN AND CARROTS
1 TABLESPOON TAHINI
100ml TOMATO PASTE
HERBS (for example, basil, oregano, marjoram, thyme, rosemary)
SPICES (for example, chilli, curry powder, mixed spice, paprika)
SALT (optional)
OIL
1 TABLESPOON NUT BUTTER (for example, cashew butter or hazelnut butter)
1 CUP COTTAGE CHEESE (low fat)
STRING BEANS

Chop onions and garlic and saute in oil until brown. Meanwhile, steam the diced sweet potato, pumpkin and carrots until soft. Mash and add a pinch of mixed spice and curry powder. Once onions are browned, add the mince and brown it.

Meanwhile, mix together the tahini, tomato paste, herbs, chilli, paprika and salt. Also add the nut butter and some water, enough to make a firm sauce.

Once the mince has browned and any excess fluid has evaporated, add the sauce and stir in well. Place in a shallow baking dish. Placed the mashed sweet potato, pumpkin and carrot on top of the mince. Sprinkle with a small amount of cottage cheese. Place in the oven at 180°C for about half an hour.

Meanwhile, prepare the spring beans and steam.
Serve the shepherd's pie with the beans and some sprouts.
Preferably have the C-Herb Tea before the meal.

> *HINT:* Left-overs from this dish make a wonderful snack for another time. Just allow it to cool and then store in the freezer. When required, allow to thaw, and then reheat.

BREAKFAST WEEK 1 DAY 5
- Muesli-porridge
- Toasted loaf (optional)
- C-Herb Tea

¾ CUP MUESLI-PORRIDGE (see Index)

350ml MILK/WATER

DESIRED NUMBER OF SLICES OF LOAF, TOASTED

SPREAD OF CHOICE

FRUIT, if allowed (fresh *not* dried)

Add the milk or water to the muesli-porridge. Bring to the boil, then simmer for 3 to 5 minutes. A knob of butter or a dash of oil can be added, once cooked. Mix in the fruit (if allowed).

Preferably have the C-Herb Tea before the meal.
Serves one.

This muesli-porridge mix can be eaten uncooked (requires a good digestive system!). Simply add hot or cold milk and eat.

MENU FOR WEEK 1: BREAKFAST, LUNCH, DINNER

LUNCH WEEK 1 DAY 5
- Meatballs and salad
- C-Herb Tea

500g VEAL MINCE (OR CHICKEN MINCE)
1 SMALL ONION
1 TABLESPOON WHOLEMEAL FLOUR
1 TABLESPOON SUNFLOWER SEEDS
1 EGG
50g FINELY DICED CAPSICUM
OIL
1 TEASPOON SESAME SEEDS
MIXED HERBS
PARSLEY
SALT/PEPPER (optional)
SPICES (for example, paprika, curry and chilli)
THERMOS OF C-HERB TEA

Place mince in a mixing bowl. Add the finely diced capsicum, onion, sunflower seeds, sesame seeds, egg, herbs, spices and flour. To mix, use fingers. Continue to squeeze and knead until well mixed. Make into 4 firm balls and fry in oil until brown.

Serve with salad. Any left-over meatballs make good snacks for later.
Preferably have the C-Herb Tea before the meal.

UNDERSTANDING CANDIDA

DINNER WEEK 1 DAY 5
- Omelette
- Silverbeet
- Damper
- C-Herb Tea

3 EGGS

1 SMALL ONION

1 SMALL CARROT

¼ CUP DICED CAPSICUM

100g EGGPLANT

¼ CUP PEAS

1 FLAT TABLESPOON BUTTER

HERBS (for example, basil, oregano, marjoram, parsley)

SPICES

SALT/PEPPER (optional)

MILK

Chop the onion and eggplant into small pieces and saute together until brown. Use sufficient oil. Finely chop the carrot and capsicum. Shell the peas. Mix with the onion and eggplant once they have browned. Set aside. Crack the eggs into a small bowl. Add the herbs and spices. Melt the butter in frypan. Whisk the eggs briskly with a dash of milk. Pour into frypan. Allow to slightly set before adding the other ingredients. Cook slowly until firm, then place under the griller to brown the top of the omelette.

Serve with hot, crusty damper (see Index) and silverbeet.

INGREDIENTS FOR SILVERBEET

4 STALKS AND LEAVES OF SILVERBEET

200ml MILK

SALT/PEPPER (optional)

MASTERFOOD'S MEXICAN STYLE CHILLI (or similar)

1 KNOB BUTTER

2 TEASPOONS WHOLEMEAL FLOUR

MIXED HERBS

Steam the silverbeet for 10 to 15 minutes. Chop finely. Mix plenty of the herbs

MENU FOR WEEK 1: BREAKFAST, LUNCH, DINNER

and spices with the milk in a pan. Bring almost to the boil. In another pan, mix the flour with sufficient milk to make a thin paste. Gently add the flour paste to the hot milk, continuously stirring until thick. Add to the chopped silverbeet leaves and stalks.

Serve with the omelette and damper.

> *HINT:* Remove portion of frozen soup from the freezer for tomorrow's breakfast.

BREAKFAST WEEK 1 DAY 6
- Hearty soup
- Toasted loaf
- C-Herb Tea

PORTION OF SOUP

DESIRED NUMBER OF SLICES OF LOAF

SPROUTS

Heat the soup. Serve with toasted loaf and sprouts.

> *HINT:* Defrost chicken mince for mince loaf tonight.

LUNCH WEEK 1 DAY 6
- Sandwiches
- Salad
- C-Herb Tea

DESIRED NUMBER OF SLICES OF LOAF

DESIRED SELECTION OF SPREADS

SALAD

THERMOS OF C-HERB TEA

Prepare the sandwiches and salad. Package separately.
 Preferably have the C-Herb Tea before the meal.

> *HINT:* Defrost chicken fillets/veal cubes for kebabs.

UNDERSTANDING CANDIDA

DINNER WEEK 1 DAY 6
- Chicken loaf
- Brown rice and savoury sauce
- Steamed pumpkin
- C-Herb Tea

750g CHICKEN MINCE
2 MEDIUM ONIONS
1 SMALL CARROT
75g CAPSICUM
SALT/PEPPER
1 EGG
MIXED HERBS
SPICES (for example, curry powder, chilli, paprika)
2 TEASPOONS SESAME SEEDS
1 TABLESPOON WHOLEMEAL FLOUR
½ CUP BROWN RICE
170g PUMPKIN
100g EGGPLANT
4 TABLESPOONS TOMATO PASTE
1 TABLESPOON TAHINI
OIL

Place the mince in a large mixing bowl. Finely chop one onion. Dice the carrot and capsicum. Add to the mince. Add the egg, herbs and spices, flour and sesame seeds. Use your fingers to mix the ingredients until well blended. Grease a bread tin with butter. Place the mince mixture in the tin. Cook in an oven at 200°C for 30 to 40 minutes. Meanwhile, boil the rice and prepare the pumpkin for steaming. Chop the remaining onion and eggplant and saute together until brown. In a separate small dish, mix the tahini and tomato paste together with enough water to make a sauce.

When the chicken loaf is cooked, remove from the tin, slice, and serve with the steamed pumpkin and rice. Pour the sauce over the rice.

Preferably have the C-Herb Tea before the meal.

> *HINT:* Keep the left-over chicken loaf for sandwiches and snacks. Prepare kebabs for tomorrow's lunch.

MENU FOR WEEK I: BREAKFAST, LUNCH, DINNER

BREAKFAST WEEK 1 DAY 7
- Fried egg on rice cakes
- C-Herb Tea

2 EGGS
OIL
DESIRED NUMBER OF RICE CAKES
SPROUTS
MIXED HERBS
SALT/PEPPER (optional)

Fry the eggs in a dash of oil. Serve on the rice cakes with some sprouts and season as desired.
    Preferably have the C-Herb Tea before the meal.
    Serves one.

UNDERSTANDING CANDIDA

LUNCH WEEK 1 DAY 7
- Chicken and veal kebab
- Salad
- Loaf or scones
- C-Herb Tea

250g DICED VEAL
2 LARGE CHICKEN BREAST FILLETS
1 CAPSICUM
1 MEDIUM ONION
KEBAB STICKS
SALT/PEPPER (optional)
HERBS (for example, rosemary, oregano)
1 TABLESPOON HAZELNUT BUTTER
1 TEASPOON TAHINI
2 TABLESPOONS TOMATO PASTE
MASTERFOODS MEXICAN STYLE CHILLI (or similar)
OIL

Cut the chicken fillets into pieces. Skewer the chicken and veal pieces alternately, with slices of capsicum and onion in between. Brush well with oil. Season with herbs and spices, except for the chilli. Place in a shallow dish on a rack, as a lot of fluid accumulates in the cooking (this can be stored to use as stock for soup). Cover with foil and place in the oven at 180°C for 40 minutes. Remove and place under griller until barbequed.

Prepare a nut sauce by mixing the hazelnut butter, tahini and tomato paste with enough water to make a sauce. Add the chilli and mix in well. Heat and serve over the kebabs.

Preferably have the C-Herb Tea before the meal.

This is a meal that is easily prepared beforehand and then grilled just before serving.

DINNER WEEK 1 DAY 7
- Stuffed capsicum
- Salad (or steamed vegetables)
- C-Herb Tea

MENU FOR WEEK I: BREAKFAST, LUNCH, DINNER

2 CAPSICUMS
2 SMALL ONIONS
250g TIN TUNA/SALMON (preferably in brine)
SALT/PEPPER (optional)
2 CLOVES GARLIC
OIL
1 MEDIUM CARROT
120g PEAS
PARSLEY
4 TABLESPOONS TOMATO PASTE
SPICES
HERBS (for example, basil, oregano, mixed herbs)
½ CUP BROWN RICE
1 HEAPED TEASPOON HAZELNUT BUTTER
1 TABLESPOON TAHINI

Boil the brown rice. Briefly boil the peas for 5 to 8 minutes. Drain and set aside. Meanwhile, chop the onions and saute until almost brown. Add the garlic and saute a little longer. Drain the fish. Add to the onions.

Choose capsicums that are flat-topped (where the end opposite the stalk is flattish) so that they can stand up on their ends. Cut out the stalk, using a small, sharp knife. As this is pulled out, the entire seed 'ball' inside should come with it, too.

Mix the hazelnut butter and tahini into a sauce with some hot water. Add this to the remaining ingredients, including the peas. Mix well.

Fill the hollow capsicums with this mixture, using a tablespoon. Wrap in foil (this prevents the capsicum from burning and turning bitter). Place on baking tray and cook in an oven at 180°C for about 45 minutes. Serve hot with a salad.

Preferably have the C-Herb Tea before the meal.

This is a meal in itself, containing the vegetable, carbohydrate and protein all in one. Serve hot or cold for tomorrow's lunch. Fresh or reheated scones can be served at the same time.

HINT: Defrost lamb chops for tomorrow's breakfast.

4 SHOPPING LIST FOR WEEK TWO

BUTCHER
- 4 Lamb chops
- 1 medium chicken
- 250g chicken mince
- 250g veal mince (see dinner choice, day 2 week 2)
- 4 chicken fillets (breast or thigh)
- 500g diced veal
- soup bones, if needed (for soup)

FISH
- 2 fish fillets

HEALTH FOOD STORE
- 1kg lentils
- 500g whole wheat
- 1kg brown rice
- 1 to 2 pkts rice cakes
- 2 to 3 loaves yeast-free bread
- 500g rice flour
- 250g bran
- 500g sunflower seeds
- 1 tin/pkt vegetarian sausages (no yeast/sugar)
- 250g hulled millet
- 500g buckwheat
- 500g rolled oats
- 500g mixed or individual nuts
- 250g pipetas
- 1 to 2 pkts biscuits (yeast/sugar free)
- 250g kouskous
- Soy milk
- 1 to 2 vanilla beans

Top up or replace supplies of:
- Buckwheat flour
- Cornmeal
- Nut butters
- Oil
- Wholemeal self-raising flour

UNDERSTANDING CANDIDA

- Tahini
- Almonds (for nut milk)
- Pure protein powder

GROCER
- 1 dozen eggs (preferably free range)
- 1 × 200g tin tuna/salmon (in oil or brine)
- 1 to 2 tins sardines (for sandwiches)

GREENGROCER
- 2 containers sprouts
- 3kg tomatoes (2kg for tomato paste)
- 3 to 4 capsicums
- 2 lettuces
- 1kg carrots
- 3 to 4 avocado
- 1 bunch radishes
- 3 medium sweet potato
- 1 large piece pumpkin
- 4 parsnips
- 2kg onions
- 1 head garlic
- 2 cucumbers
- 2 bunches chives
- 6 medium zucchini
- 100g ginger
- 2 bunches parsley
- 10 lemons
- 1 large eggplant
- ½ cabbage
- 100g peas
- ¼ cauliflower
- 500g green beans
- 1 small bunch beetroot
- 1 head broccoli

5 MENU FOR WEEK TWO: BREAKFAST, LUNCH, DINNER

BREAKFAST WEEK 2 DAY 1
- Grilled lamb chops, tomato and sprouts
- Buckwheat and corn pikelets
- C-Herb Tea

<u>**2 LAMB CHOPS (remove as much fat as possible)**</u>
½ TOMATO

SPROUTS

SPREADS

BUCKWHEAT AND CORN PIKELETS (see Index)

While the pikelets are cooking, grill 2 chops. Also place ½ tomato under the griller.

Serve together with the pikelets, which can be topped with a variety of spreads. Finish off with a tuft of sprouts.

Preferably have the C-Herb Tea before the meal.

Serves one.

LUNCH WEEK 2 DAY 1
- Stuffed capsicum
- Salad
- C-Herb Tea

SEE * OR SIMPLY REHEAT THE SPARE CAPSICUM FROM YESTERDAY

Thermos C-Herb Tea

* Dinner, Day 7, Week 1.

DINNER WEEK 2 DAY 1
- Baked chicken and vegetables
- Salad or steamed vegetables
- C-Herb Tea

1 × SIZE 10 CHICKEN
OIL
2 × 125g PIECE OF SWEET POTATO AND PUMPKIN
2 SMALL PARSNIPS
2 SMALL ONIONS
SPICES
SALT (optional)
MIXED HERBS
SALAD OR SELECTION OF STEAMED VEGETABLES
CHILLI

Brush the chicken with the oil and sprinkle with salt, chilli and mixed herbs. Place 2 to 3 pinches of allspice into the belly of the chicken.

Brush sweet potato, pumpkin, parsnip and onion with oil and place in the bottom of a baking tray. Position the chicken on a rack, above the vegetables. Place in an oven at 180°C for a total of 1½ hours. After 45 minutes turn the chicken and baste the vegetables.

Prepare the salad or steam the vegetables just before chicken is ready to serve.

Preferably have the C-Herb Tea before the meal.

> *HINT:* Store left-over chicken in the fridge for tomorrow's lunch. Defrost fish for tomorrow's breakfast.

MENU FOR WEEK II: BREAKFAST, LUNCH, DINNER

BREAKFAST WEEK 2 DAY 2
- Fish (grilled or baked)
- Toasted loaf or scones
- C-Herb Tea

1 PIECE OF FISH FILLET

2 SLICES TOMATO

SALT (optional)

DILL (small pinch)

KNOB OF BUTTER (optional)

1 SMALL ONION

1 CLOVE GARLIC (optional)

SPROUTS

2 SLICES CUCUMBER

Lightly salt the fish fillet. Place in casserole dish or on foil. Sprinkle the dill, onions and garlic over the fish. Place slices of tomato on top with knob of butter. Close the foil or cover the casserole dish and place in the oven at 200°C for 20 to 25 minutes.
   Serve with sprouts, cucumber, toast or scones (reheated from freezer).
   Preferably have the C-Herb Tea before the meal.
   Serves one.

> HINT: Soak lentils or defrost mince for dinner tonight.

LUNCH WEEK 2 DAY 2
- Cold chicken
- Salad
- Wholemeal scones
- C-Herb Tea

¼ CHICKEN PIECE, LEG OR BREAST PORTION, COLD

SALAD

DESIRED NUMBER OF WHOLEMEAL SCONES

THERMOS OF C-HERB TEA

The chicken piece could be left over from yesterday's dinner. Wrap the scones in foil and place in the oven at 220°C for 15 minutes. Serve hot with the chicken and the salad.

Preferably have the C-Herb Tea before the meal.

DINNER WEEK 2 DAY 2
- Moussaka
- Steamed vegetables or salad
- C-Herb Tea

1 MEDIUM ONION
350g EGGPLANT
¾ CUP LENTILS (A 1:1 CHICKEN-VEAL MINCE MIXTURE COULD BE USED INSTEAD)
OIL
2 CLOVES GARLIC
½ CUP WHOLE WHEAT (OR BROWN RICE)
½ CUP TOMATO PASTE
1 CARROT
SALT/PEPPER (optional)
1 TABLESPOON TAHINI
MIXED HERBS
SPICES (for example, paprika, curry powder, chilli)
SELECTION OF VEGETABLES FOR STEAMING

Presoak or quick-soak the lentils. Cook for 5 minutes. Cut the eggplant into thin slices. Fry in the oil until brown on both sides. Place aside. Chop the onions and garlic and saute until brown. Add the lentils (or brown the mince, if using the alternative ingredient).

In a separate pan, mix together the tomato paste, tahini, herbs and spices and enough water to make a sauce. Add to the onions and lentils or mince. Mix well. Place a layer of the fried eggplant slices on the bottom of the casserole dish and alternately add further layers of the lentils, carrot slices and eggplant. Cover casserole dish. Place in the oven at 180°C for about 45 minutes.

Meanwhile, cook the whole wheat or brown rice (see Index). Serve with the steamed vegetables or salad.

Preferably have the C-Herb Tea before the meal.

HINT: Keep the left-overs for lunch tomorrow.

MENU FOR WEEK II: BREAKFAST, LUNCH, DINNER

BREAKFAST WEEK 2 DAY 3
- Scrambled eggs and tomato
- Rice cakes
- C-Herb Tea

2 EGGS
MILK
1 SMALL ONION
CHIVES/PARSLEY/OREGANO
¼ CUP DICED CAPSICUM
¼ CUP DICED ZUCCHINI
OIL
SALT/PEPPER (optional)
1 TO 2 TEASPOONS TOMATO PASTE
1 CLOVE GARLIC
1 TO 2 RICE CAKES
½ TOMATO
SPROUTS

Chop the onion and garlic and saute in oil until brown. Add the diced capsicum and zucchini, the tomato paste, herbs, salt, pepper, a dash of milk. Add the eggs and stir well until cooked. Serve on rice cakes with a grilled half tomato and some sprouts.
   Preferably have the C-Herb Tea before the meal.
   Serves one.

LUNCH WEEK 2 DAY 3
- Moussaka
- Scones or toasted loaf
- C-Herb Tea
- Salad

MOUSSAKA (from yesterday's dinner)
WHOLEMEAL SCONES (previously made)
THERMOS OF C-HERB TEA
SALAD

Reheat the moussaka and the scones. Serve with a salad.
   Preferably have the C-Herb Tea before the meal.

DINNER WEEK 2 DAY 3
- Fish cakes
- Salad or steamed vegetables
- Damper
- C-Herb Tea

1 CUP COOKED, FLAKED FISH (OR TINNED SALMON/TUNA)
1 TABLESPOON FINELY CHOPPED ONION
1 TEASPOON GRATED GINGER ROOT
1 TABLESPOON CHOPPED PARSLEY
PINCH OF NUTMEG AND CAYENNE PEPPER
SALT/PEPPER (optional)
1 TABLESPOON LEMON JUICE
1 CLOVE GARLIC
PINCH OF DILL
½ TEASPOON LEMON RIND
2 HEAPED TABLESPOONS RICE FLOUR
MILK
OIL
BRAN
SELECTION OF VEGETABLES FOR STEAMING

Finely chop the onion and garlic. Add all the ingredients except for the oil and bran. Mix well with sufficient milk to make the mixture into a thick paste. Make into small patties and roll in bran. Fry in some oil until brown on both sides. Makes 4 fish cakes.

Prepare the damper (see Index). Serve the fish cakes, hot damper and salad or steamed vegetables together.

Preferably have the C-Herb Tea before the meal.

MENU FOR WEEK II: BREAKFAST, LUNCH, DINNER

BREAKFAST WEEK 2 DAY 4
- Pancakes and spreads
- C-Herb Tea

Make the pancakes and use a selection of spreads (see Index).
Preferably have the C-Herb Tea before the meal.

> HINT: Soak lentils for lunch tomorrow. Defrost ingredients for the mixed grill.

LUNCH WEEK 2 DAY 4
- Sandwiches
- Salad
- C-Herb Tea

DESIRED NUMBER OF SLICES OF LOAF
CHOICE OF SPREADS
SALAD
THERMOS OF C-HERB TEA

Prepare the sandwiches and salad. Package separately.
Preferably have the C-Herb Tea before the meal.

UNDERSTANDING CANDIDA

DINNER WEEK 2 DAY 4
- Mixed grill
- Stir-fried vegetables
- Brown rice and millet
- C-Herb Tea

2 LAMB CHOPS (as lean as possible)

2 VEGETARIAN SAUSAGES (*always* check labels for yeast in such products)

2 CHICKEN FILLETS (THIGH OR BREAST)

1 MEDIUM ONION

1 ZUCCHINI

1 CARROT

1 TOMATO

1 CLOVE GARLIC

½ SMALL EGGPLANT

OIL

½ CUP TOMATO PASTE

150g CABBAGE

150g CAPSICUM

HERBS (for example, oregano, marjoram, rosemary)

SPICES (for example, paprika, cayenne pepper)

½ CUP BROWN RICE

¼ CUP MILLET (HULLED)

Sprinkle some herbs on the chops, fillets and sausages. Place under the griller and cook.

Chop the onions, garlic and eggplant. Saute together until brown. Chop the remaining vegetables and add. Keep stirring until they begin to soften. Add the tomato paste and the herbs and spices. Mix well.

Meanwhile, bring the rice to the boil. Simmer for 20 minutes, or so. As the rice is starting to soften and cook, add the millet. Keep simmering until the grains are cooked and the water is absorbed and evaporated.

Serve the stir-fried vegetables over the grains, with the grill.

Preferably have the C-Herb Tea before the meal.

> HINT: Soak the buckwheat for tomorrow's porridge. Prepare tomorrow's lunch now, if convenient.

MENU FOR WEEK II: BREAKFAST, LUNCH, DINNER

BREAKFAST WEEK 2 DAY 5
- Buckwheat and rolled oats porridge
- Boiled egg
- C-Herb Tea

40g ROLLED OATS (or any rolled/'flaked' grain)
20g BUCKWHEAT
450ml WATER
KNOB OF BUTTER OR 1 TO 2 TEASPOONS OIL
CINNAMON/NUTMEG
1 TEASPOON ROASTED SESAME SEEDS (optional)
1 TO 2 EGGS, AS DESIRED

Soak the buckwheat overnight in the 450ml of water. Bring to the boil. Add the rolled oats. Simmer very slowly for 5 to 10 minutes. Before serving, add cinnamon and mix in well.

Finally, add the butter or oil and sprinkle with the roasted sesame seeds. These can be freshly roasted by placing in a heavy, unoiled frypan. Heat and stir the sesame seeds until golden brown. Prepare only as much as you would use in a week's cooking.

Boil the egg(s) to the desired hardness.
Preferably have the C-Herb Tea before the meal.
Serves one.

> *HINT:* Soak lentils for dinner tonight.

UNDERSTANDING CANDIDA

LUNCH WEEK 2 DAY 5
- Savoury lentils and rice
- Salad
- C-Herb Tea

½ CUP LENTILS
¼ CUP BROWN RICE
OIL
1 TO 2 CLOVES GARLIC
1 FLAT TEASPOON GRATED GINGER
1 CUP TOMATO PASTE
CURRY POWDER (as much as desired)
100g PEAS
MASTERFOODS MEXICAN STYLE CHILLI (or similar)
1 SMALL CARROT
SALT/PEPPER (optional)
HERBS (for example, oregano, basil, rosemary)
PAPRIKA
1 MEDIUM ONION

Presoak or 'quick soak' lentils. Rinse well. Bring to the boil. Simmer for about 15 minutes. Boil brown rice. Boil the peas.

Meanwhile, chop the onion and garlic and saute in oil until brown. Add the ginger, tomato paste, finely diced carrot, cooked peas, herbs and spices. Mix well.

Combine the cooked rice and lentils. Mix gently with all the other ingredients. Serve hot, with a salad.

Preferably have the C-Herb Tea before the meal.

HINT: This dish can be frozen or stored for later use as a snack.

MENU FOR WEEK II: BREAKFAST, LUNCH, DINNER

DINNER WEEK 2 DAY 5
- Ratatouille
- Brown rice
- C-Herb Tea

350g EGGPLANT
1 LARGE ONION
150g CARROT
75g CAPSICUM
1 SMALL TOMATO
75g SWEET POTATO
½ CUP LENTILS
½ CUP BROWN RICE
OIL
WHOLEMEAL FLOUR (enough to dust the eggplant slices)
SALT/PEPPER (optional)
½ CUP TOMATO PASTE
SPICES
HERBS (for example, basil, mixed herbs, oregano)
1 TEASPOON SESAME SEEDS

Soak lentils overnight, or 'quick soak' them in very hot water for about one hour. Slice the eggplant thinly and dust in flour. Add plenty of oil to a frypan. Fry until brown on both sides.

Combine the spices, herbs, sesame seeds and salt, with the soaked lentils. Line the bottom of the casserole dish with a layer of eggplant. Next, mix together the sliced sweet potato, carrot, onion, capsicum, tomato and lentils. Make alternative layers, finishing with a layer of fried eggplant slices. Cover and place in the oven at 150°C for about 1 ½ hours.

Boil the brown rice in about 400ml of water. Allow to simmer for about 25 minutes, until the water has evaporated and the grain is cooked (this may take a bit of juggling for the first few times; in fact, it is not hard to achieve).

Serve the ratatouille over the boiled brown rice and add some sprouts.

Preferably have the C-Herb Tea before the meal.

UNDERSTANDING CANDIDA

BREAKFAST WEEK 2 DAY 6
- Mixed nuts and seeds
- Wholemeal scones or loaf toast
- Sprouts
- C-Herb Tea

DESIRED AMOUNT OF NUTS AND SEEDS
WHOLEMEAL SCONES OR LOAF
SPROUTS
SPREADS

Select nuts and seeds. Either toast desired number of slices of loaf or heat the scones by wrapping them in foil and placing them in the oven at 220°C for about 15 minutes. Top with desired selection of spreads. Serve with some added sprouts.

> HINT: Defrost the fish for dinner tonight.

LUNCH WEEK 2 DAY 6
- Ratatouille
- Salad
- Biscuits (yeast/sugar free)
- C-Herb Tea

RATATOUILLE FROM LAST NIGHT
SALAD
DESIRED NUMBER OF BISCUITS
THERMOS OF C-HERB TEA

Package ratatouille and salad separately. Reheat ratatouille. Butter the biscuits in advance.
   Preferably have the C-Herb Tea before the meal.

MENU FOR WEEK II: BREAKFAST, LUNCH, DINNER

DINNER WEEK 2 DAY 6
- Fish
- Steamed vegetables (or salad)
- Kouskous
- C-Herb Tea

1 FISH FILLET (any type)

KNOB OF BUTTER

OIL

RANGE OF VEGETABLES (for example, 1 small carrot, 1 small zucchini, 1 small piece of cauliflower)

1 SMALL TOMATO

¼ CUP KOUSKOUS (from health food stores)

TOMATO PASTE

HERBS (for example, dill, basil, oregano)

TAHINI

1 SMALL ONION

SALT/PEPPER

Place the fillet of fish into a casserole dish or onto a sheet of foil. Cover the fish with slices of tomato. Sprinkle with the herbs and seasoning as desired. Add a knob of butter. Close the foil or cover the casserole dish. Place in the oven at 200°C for about 30 minutes.

Meanwhile, chop the onion and saute until brown in the oil. Add the tomato paste and 1 tablespoon of tahini to the onions. Thin with some water. Mix well into a thin sauce. Add basil and oregano.

Prepare the vegetables and steam.

Boil about 1 litre of water. Add ¼ cup kouskous. Simmer for about 3 to 5 minutes. Drain and serve with the fish and vegetables. Pour the sauce over the kouskous.

Preferably have the C-Herb Tea before the meal.
Serves one.

HINT: Defrost chicken fillet for tomorrow's breakfast.

BREAKFAST WEEK 2 DAY 7
- Fried/grilled chicken breast fillet
- Toasted loaf
- Sprouts
- C-Herb Tea

1 TO 2 CHICKEN BREAST FILLETS (or thigh fillets)
1 TABLESPOON OIL
1 TO 2 TABLESPOONS TOMATO PASTE
DESIRED NUMBER OF SLICES OF TOASTED LOAF
2 SLICES OF CUCUMBER
SPROUTS

If grilling the fillets, place under grill until cooked. If frying, heat oil in frypan and add chicken fillets. Cover. Fry until cooked. When done, add the tomato paste. Heat briefly before serving with the toast, cucumber and sprouts.

Preferably have the C-Herb Tea before the meal.
Serves one.

> HINT: Defrost veal for dinner tonight.

LUNCH WEEK 2 DAY 7
- Boiled eggs
- Salad
- Rice cakes
- C-Herb Tea

1 TO 2 EGGS
SALAD
DESIRED NUMBER OF RICE CAKES
THERMOS OF C-HERB TEA
SPREADS

Hard boil the eggs. Butter the rice cakes and top with desired spreads. Prepare and pack your choice of salad.

Preferably have the C-Herb Tea before the meal.

MENU FOR WEEK II: BREAKFAST, LUNCH, DINNER

DINNER WEEK 2 DAY 7
- Veal casserole
- Brown rice
- Steamed vegetables
- C-Herb Tea

1 MEDIUM ONION
500g DICED VEAL
SALT/PEPPER (optional)
2 TABLESPOONS WHOLEMEAL FLOUR
1 FLAT TEASPOON PAPRIKA
HERBS (for example, basil, parsley, rosemary)
1 MEDIUM TOMATO
1 CAPSICUM
2 CLOVES GARLIC
3 TABLESPOONS TOMATO PASTE
100ml WATER
½ CUP BROWN RICE
PUMPKIN AND BEANS (quantities as desired)

Chop the onions and saute until brown. Mix the herbs and spices with the flour in a plastic bag. Add the diced veal. Seal the plastic bag, leaving plenty of air inside. Toss vigorously until the veal pieces are well coated. Add to the onions and briefly stir fry.

Chop the garlic, tomato and capsicum. Stir in with the veal. Place in crockpot or casserole dish. Mix the 100ml of water with the tomato paste and pour over contents in the crockpot. Cook at a low setting for 8 to 10 hours or place in the oven at 180°C for about 2 hours.

Serve with boiled brown rice and steamed vegetables.
Preferably take the C-Herb Tea before the meal.

HINT: This recipe will provide 2 to 3 servings, so freeze left-overs for snacks that can quickly be reheated at any time. Prepare chicken legs for tomorrow's breakfast and salad for tomorrow's lunch, if necessary.

6 SALADS, SNACK FOODS, SAUCES...AND MORE!

GREEN SALAD

1 SMALL TOMATO

150g CUCUMBER

85g ZUCCHINI

½ STALK CELERY

85g CAPSICUM

¾ CUP SPROUTS

60g BEETROOT (cubed, steamed and cooled)

1 HEAPED TABLESPOON CHOPPED CHIVES

80g CABBAGE

120g LETTUCE

1 MEDIUM CARROT

1 SPRIG PARSLEY

2 TABLESPOONS SUNFLOWER SEEDS

2 TEASPOONS SESAME SEEDS

Chop or grate all the ingredients. Place in a large plastic leak-proof bag. Pour in the salad dressing. Seal the top of the bag. Shake well. Place in a bowl and serve.

The suggested proportions of ingredients are a rough guide only and provide enough for at least 4 servings. Experiment as much as you wish.

UNDERSTANDING CANDIDA

GREEN AND RED SALAD

120g LETTUCE

120g RED CAPSICUM

1 MEDIUM TOMATO

1 MEDIUM CARROT

150g CABBAGE

1 VERY SMALL ONION

1 TABLESPOON FINELY CHOPPED FRESH BASIL

1 TABLESPOON FINELY CHOPPED PARSLEY

150g BEETROOT (cubed, steamed and cooled)

Grate or chop the ingredients. Place in a large plastic bag. Make a salad dressing (see Index), and pour contents in the bag. Seal the top of bag and shake well to mix. Enough for about 3 to 4 servings.

MACARONI-NUT SALAD

200g LETTUCE

80g CAPSICUM

½ STICK CELERY

1 SMALL TOMATO

2 TABLESPOONS FINELY CHOPPED CHIVES

150g CUCUMBER

100g CRUSHED MIXED NUTS

2 CUPS WHOLEMEAL MACARONI

SALAD DRESSING

Cook the macaroni until soft (don't overcook). Strain and cool. Meanwhile, chop, shred or slice the other ingredients. Place in a large plastic bag, with the cooled macaroni. Pour in a salad dressing of your choice. Seal the top of the bag and shake the contents well, mixing thoroughly. Enough for about 3 to 4 servings.

SALADS, SNACK FOODS, SAUCES AND MORE!

QUICKIE SALAD

CARROT

CUCUMBER

TOMATO

CELERY

CAPSICUM

LETTUCE

RADISH

ZUCCHINI

SPROUTS

BEETROOT (cooked at home)

AVOCADO

ENDIVE

Cut into pieces any one or more from the selection of ingredients. Place in a container to take to work. No grating, slicing, mixing necessary: so easy!

SALAD DRESSING

Below is an example of a salad dressing you can make. The proportions are up to you, depending on the preferences of your palate (salty, spicy or hot). With the herbs and spices, start off with perhaps a pinch of each. One basic rule for making a plain salad dressing is to follow a ratio of 2:1 of oil and lemon juice. Using that as a basis, you can then go on to make any number of variations by adding different herbs and spices. Remember to record the ingredients as you experiment!

50ml OIL

25ml LEMON JUICE

¼ TEASPOON DRY MUSTARD POWDER

SALT/PEPPER

1 TEASPOON TOMATO PASTE

1 CLOVE GARLIC

HERBS (for example, rosemary, oregano, marjoram)

SPICES

Place all the ingredients in a small jar. Seal well. Shake thoroughly. Can be stored in the fridge for several days. Shake again before serving.

GINGER SAUCE

1 LARGE ONION
1 CLOVE GARLIC
50g FRESH GINGER ROOT
OIL
1 TEASPOON TAHINI
2 TABLESPOONS LEMON JUICE

Chop the onions and garlic and saute in oil until brown. Add finely chopped or grated ginger root, tahini and water to make a sauce of the desired consistency.
 This sauce goes very well with fish dishes.

TAHINI SAUCE

1 CLOVE GARLIC
PINCH SALT
½ CUP LEMON JUICE
½ CUP TAHINI
1 TABLESPOON OIL
HERBS (for example, coriander, dill, basil, oregano)

Crush garlic. Add salt, oil and lemon juice. Mix in the herbs. Gradually add the tahini, mixing continually until the desired thickness is achieved. This will keep for several days in tightly sealed containers in the refrigerator.
 This sauce goes very well with many dishes and can be used with steamed vegetables or boiled rice to add more flavour.

SALADS, SNACK FOODS, SAUCES AND MORE!

LENTIL SOUP

2kg SOUP BONES
2 CUPS LENTILS
2 LARGE ONIONS
150g PARSNIP
150g SWEET POTATO
2 SMALL CARROTS
SALT/PEPPER (optional)
HERBS (for example, parsley, bay leaf, rosemary, oregano)
MASTERFOODS MEXICAN STYLE CHILLI (or similar)
CURRY POWDER
2 TO 3 CLOVES GARLIC

Soak the lentils overnight. Rinse well. Boil the soup bones for about one hour before removing them. Once the stock has cooled, the solidified fat can be very easily skimmed off. Add the soaked and rinsed lentils to the stock. Bring to a simmer. Meanwhile, chop then saute the onions and garlic until brown. Add to the stock with the chopped parsnips, sweet potato and carrots.

Simmer with lid on for about one more hour, stirring every now and then. When a soup consistency has been reached, take off the heat. Add all the herbs and spices. Mix in well and let stand.

This soup can be easily frozen and kept as a snack or a meal for another time.

CHICKEN SOUP

1 × SIZE 10 CHICKEN
1 MEDIUM PARSNIP
1 MEDIUM CARROT
1 MEDIUM ZUCCHINI
1 MEDIUM BEETROOT
2 LARGE ONIONS
150g STRING BEANS
3 LITRES WATER
1 SMALL CAPSICUM
150g PUMPKIN
1 SMALL TOMATO
4 TABLESPOONS OIL
SALT (optional)
HERBS (for example, bay leaf)
SPICES (for example, paprika, curry)

Remove the skin from the chicken. Place chicken in the water in a large pan. Bring to the boil. Simmer for about 1 hour.

Meanwhile, chop up the onions. Saute in the oil until brown. Set aside. Chop and prepare the vegetables.

After 1 hour, remove the chicken from the stock. Allow to cool. Add the vegetables and sauted onions to the stock. Once the chicken has cooled, remove the meat from the bones, cut to size and return to the stock. Allow to simmer for another 30 minutes. Whole wheat grains, brown rice, any other grains or wholemeal pasta can be added to the stock now. Add herbs and spices. Stir in well. Allow to cool before placing into plastic containers for freezing.

Similar stocks and soups can be made using these ingredients: instead of chicken, use lamb shanks, beef spare ribs, ox tongue or soup bones.

SALADS, SNACK FOODS, SAUCES AND MORE!

SPREADS

AVOCADO

NUT BUTTERS (for example, cashew or hazel nut. Peanut butter in small amounts, only if tolerated)

TUNA/SALMON/SARDINES (in oil or brine)

COLD CHICKEN (chopped or sliced)

COLD MEAT LOAF OR CHICKEN LOAF (see Index)

COLD, BOILED LIVER (lamb's liver is best), SLICED. Sounds hideous but is actually very nice and nutritious

SUNFLOWER SEEDS (whole or as paste)

TOMATO/LETTUCE/ONIONS/SPROUTS/CUCUMBER

TAHINI

TUNA SPREAD (see Index)

AVOCADO SPREAD (see Index)

LENTIL SPREAD (see Index)

SLICED, COOKED OX TONGUE

This list can only be exhausted and limited by your own imagination.

TUNA SPREAD

1 × 170g TIN TUNA (in oil or brine), DRAINED

250g COTTAGE CHEESE

1 TABLESPOON TAHINI

1 TABLESPOON FRESH CHIVES, FINELY CHOPPED

PINCH CAYENNE PEPPER

½ TEASPOON SALT (optional)

40g TOFU

PINCH DILL

PINCH ROSEMARY

2 TEASPOONS LEMON JUICE

Mix all the ingredients very well until a smooth paste has been formed. Use on slices of loaf, crackers and Ryvita.

Store in sealed containers in the fridge. Will keep for several days.

LENTIL SPREAD

½ CUP CHICKPEAS
½ CUP LENTILS
½ LEMON
2 TO 3 CLOVES GARLIC
½ TEASPOON CURRY POWDER
SALT/PEPPER
½ TEASPOON CHOPPED CHIVES
1 TABLESPOON OIL
½ TABLESPOON FINELY CHOPPED PARSLEY
½ CUP TAHINI
MIXED HERBS/SPICES

Soak the chickpeas and lentils overnight. Cook until quite soft (about 30 to 40 minutes). Drain well. Add lemon juice and all the other ingredients. Mash well into a paste. Use as a spread. Refrigerate. Will keep for at least 4 to 5 days.

AVOCADO SPREAD

2 RIPE AVOCADO
1 RIPE TOMATO
2 TABLESPOONS LEMON JUICE
1 TABLESPOON FINELY CHOPPED CHIVES
1 CRUSHED CLOVE GARLIC
½ TEASPOON DRIED BASIL
PINCH CAYENNE PEPPER
40g TOFU
SALT/PEPPER

Peel the tomato (made easier by briefly placing in boiling water). Chop finely. Place in the bottom of the blender. Add the herbs and spices. Add the lemon juice and, finally, the scooped out avocado. Blend to a firm paste. Refrigerate. Should keep for at least 3 to 5 days. This is a recipe where you may add more herbs and spices if you really like savoury things.

NUT MILK

Nut milk is very nutritious, palatable and extremely easy to make. It is best to prepare only one to two days' supply at a time and always refrigerate like normal milk. Before serving, mix the milk briefly, for a more even consistency.

SALADS, SNACK FOODS, SAUCES AND MORE!

The ground remains of the nuts, after they have been squeezed for their milk, should not be wasted. This is a high protein food and can be added to gravies, sauces, soups or stews. Mixed in with some tahini, it goes well as a spread for sandwiches, pikelets and scones.

Experiment with your own combination and choice of nuts and seeds and change the ratio of water and solids, as desired. Various spices such as cinnamon, nutmeg or a vanilla bean can be used to enhance the flavour.

Below are three basic recipes that give you some idea of the proportions that work (but experiment as much as you would like).

1. 100g ALMONDS
   2 CUPS WATER
2. 30g SESAME SEEDS (you may also roast them)
   30g SUNFLOWER SEEDS
   40g ALMONDS
3. 50g ALMONDS
   50g SUNFLOWER SEEDS
   1 HEAPED TEASPOON SOY FLOUR

For each combination, place the ingredients into a blender and blend for a good 2 minutes. Strain through a fine-weave cloth (a tea towel), and wring out as much milk as possible.

TOMATO PASTE

3 LARGE ONIONS

1 LARGE RED CAPSICUM

6 CLOVES GARLIC

OIL

2kg RIPE TOMATOES

3 BAY LEAVES

1 HEAPED TEASPOON BASIL

½ TEASPOON OREGANO

½ TEASPOON MARJORAM

SALT/PEPPER (optional)

½ TEASPOON CHILLI

PINCH OF CURRY

½ TEASPOON PAPRIKA

¼ TEASPOON ROSEMARY (powdered)

PINCH OF MIXED SPICE

1 TABLESPOON PARSLEY

½ TEASPOON DRY MUSTARD POWDER

NOTE: *This recipe takes very little effort, but quite some time: choose your opportunity wisely!*

Finely chop the onions and garlic and saute in plenty of oil, until brown.

Cut the tomatoes and capsicum. Puree together in a blender. Add to the sauted onions. Bring to the boil. Simmer very slowly until reduced to a paste-like consistency.

Add the herbs and spices while still hot. Mix in well. Cover and allow to cool.

Place in containers and store in the freezer until needed.

SALADS, SNACK FOODS, SAUCES AND MORE!

MUESLI-PORRIDGE

600g ROLLED OATS (or rolled wheat/rye/rice/triticale)
3 HEAPED TABLESPOONS PURE PROTEIN POWDER (no added sugars/yeasts/starches)
100g FLAXSEED
30g ROASTED SESAME SEEDS
100g SUNFLOWER SEEDS
100g PIPETAS (pumpkin seeds)
150g CRUSHED NUTS
50g BRAN AND/OR WHEAT GERM
1 TEASPOON CINNAMON
PINCH OF MIXED SPICE
60g HULLED MILLET

NOTE: *These quantities can be increased or decreased at your discretion. This is one recipe that is an experimenter's delight!*

Place all the ingredients into a large plastic bag. Seal the top, trapping plenty of air. Shake and mix the ingredients thoroughly. Store in airtight jars or containers.

DIRECTIONS FOR EATING

Unless you have superb digestive powers (and most people with Candida do *not*), it is very difficult for your stomach to handle a combination of raw grains, especially for example millet and rolled oats. Simply add hot or cold milk to the muesli and see how your stomach handles it. It supplies a good amount of both protein and complex carbohydrate. Therefore, it can be seen as a meal in itself, especially for example millet and rolled oats. You could try simply adding hot or cold milk to the muesli and see how your stomach handles it, but it would be best to either add hot or cold milk or water the night before, let it soak and then eating it. Or you could add the water or milk in the morning, bring to the boil, simmer for about 5 mins. and serve as a very nutritious and different type of porridge. It supplies a good amount of both protein and complex carbohydrate. Therefore, it can be seen as a meal in itself, especially handy for breakfasts, or snacks during the day.

To give more flavour, particularly in the period before you are allowed fruit, you can also add a knob of butter or, preferably, a good dash of oil. This will also settle the appetite for those of you who suffer constant feelings of hunger.

Once fresh fruit is allowed by your practitioner, the appropriate amount may be chopped up and added to this muesli for flavour and sweetness.

DAMPER

2½ CUPS WHOLEMEAL SELF-RAISING FLOUR

½ CUP GLUTEN FLOUR (*only* when sure that you're not allergic to it)

1 TEASPOON BAKING POWDER

SALT

MIXED HERBS

¾ CUP WATER

¾ CUP MILK

Mix the flours, baking powder, salt and herbs together. Mix the water and milk together. Pour into the dry ingredients. Stir well to form a soft dough. Knead the dough for about 5 minutes before placing it on to a greased baking tray. Cover loosely with some foil.

Place in the oven at 150°C for 15 minutes. Then, increase the heat to 200°C. Remove the foil and bake for another 30 minutes or until crisp and brown.

Serve hot. Cool before wrapping in plastic and freezing. It can later be wrapped in foil and placed in a hot oven for 20 to 30 minutes to make it as good as freshly baked damper.

BUCKWHEAT AND CORN PIKELETS

½ CUP BUCKWHEAT FLOUR

½ CUP CORNMEAL (fine ground)

1½ CUPS MILK OR WATER

PINCH OF SALT (optional)

PINCH OF MIXED SPICE

½ TEASPOON CINNAMON

Mix the dry ingredients together. Use either entirely milk or entirely water, or make a mix of the two. Add to the flours. Beat in well to a smooth, thin consistency. Add more fluid if necessary. Let it stand for 10 minutes or so. Add further fluid, if necessary, before frying in butter or ghee, making small pikelets. Use butter: the pikelets don't stick to the pan as much as if oil were used.

Serve hot or freeze for later use.

SALADS, SNACK FOODS, SAUCES AND MORE!

SCONES

2 CUPS SELF-RAISING WHOLEMEAL FLOUR

½ CUP GLUTEN FLOUR (if not allergic to grains/gluten)

2 LEVEL TEASPOONS BAKING POWDER

PINCH SALT

1 TABLESPOON OIL

1½ CUPS MILK

¼ CUP WATER

Mix all the dry ingredients together. Heat the milk, water and oil together, before adding to the dry ingredients. Mix well into a soft dough. Roll out on floured board to about a 2cm thickness. Cut out pieces with a glass jar or a cup or with a special cutter. Place dough on a greased baking tray.

Let them stand in a warm place for 10 minutes or so, to help the rising process. Bake in oven at 200°C for 20 minutes or until browned.

Serve hot, or cool before freezing. To reheat them, wrap them in foil and place in the oven at 200°C for 15 to 20 minutes. Unwrap and serve, fresh as new!

PANCAKES

1 CUP WHOLEMEAL FLOUR

PINCH OF SALT

PINCH OF MIXED SPICE

1 EGG

1½ CUP MILK

BUTTER

Mix the dry ingredients together. Add the egg to the milk. Beat well. Add this to the flour mix and beat vigorously until a thin batter is reached. Extra milk can be used if necessary.

Melt the butter in the frypan (oil causes sticking to the pan). Pour in the batter until the bottom of the pan is thinly coated. Cook both sides until brown.

UNDERSTANDING CANDIDA

PROTEIN DRINK
½ CUP MILK
½ CUP WATER
1 HEAPED TEASPOON PROTEIN POWDER (no sugars, yeasts)
FLAVOURING (for example, nutmeg, cinnamon, vanilla bean)
1 TEASPOON PURE CAROB POWDER
1 EGG YOLK
FRUIT (when allowed)

Mix the ingredients in the blender or with a handbeater. Can be made, chilled and taken to work in a thermos.

NUTS AND SEEDS
- Hazelnuts
- Walnuts
- Brazil nuts
- Pine nuts
- Almonds
- Cashews
- Macadamian nuts
- Pecans
- Chestnuts
- Sunflower seeds
- Sesame seeds
- Pumpkin seeds (pipetas)
- Poppy seeds
- Linseed

SNACKS
For that moment in the day when you must have a snack! The list may be forever extended.
- Mixed nuts and seeds
- Sandwiches with various spreads
- Wholemeal scones and spreads
- Ryvitas or rice cakes with spreads
- Freshly popped corn (only the occasional small amount)
- Protein drink
- Chicken wings/legs
- Hard-boiled egg

SALADS, SNACK FOODS, SAUCES AND MORE!

- Quiche (left-over)
- Soup/stew (pre-made and frozen)
- Any previous meal left-overs

EPILOGUE

In our typical Western way of doing things, we make healing such a complicated business. It should be very simple. We constantly search outside the self for the source of our healing, but the truth that we so desperately search for lies within us. All we need is an awareness and the guidelines to nurture and stimulate this healing force into vibrant, health-giving action.

As each year in practice rolls by, I become more and more convinced that I cannot heal anyone, only they are able to *allow* that healing force to awaken. All I can be is a mirror and a guide. A mirror, so that each person who comes to me might see themselves a little more clearly, understanding a bit more where they might have become stuck. A guide, because all I can do is point in the direction I feel is the way of their journey. As they then walk along that path, so the healing occurs within.

I hope that this book has served as a mirror and a guide to you. The brightness with which that mirror reflects depends on many factors, both within me and within you, and some will see more clearly than others.

May each person take from the 'mirror' what they will, and may you always find the strength inside to take not only the first step on the path of healing, but all others that follow in journeying, until true, full health is attained. Ultimately, this will depend on where your own inner guide "leads you" . . .

APPENDIX

* The alpha/theta cassette can be purchased from:

Australia
- "Mystic Trader"
  Locked bag 1
  Toorak. Victoria 3142. Tel: (03) 819 6411.

- "Essential Energies"
  16 Glebe Point Rd.
  Glebe. NSW 2037. Tel: (02) 660 7008.

USA
- "Mystic Trader"
  Box 2496
  Cour d'Alene. IDAHO. USA 83814. Tel: 1-208-772-3451.

UK
- "Mystic Trader"
  Studio B
  Haverstock Hill.
  London. NW3. Tel: (01) 586 2738.

* **The M.E. Society** (for people with Myoencephalomyelitis or Post-viral Syndrome).

Australia
- PO Box 645
  Mona Vale. NSW 2103

USA
- "Chronic Fatigue & Immune Dysfunction Syndrome Association"
  Community Health Services
  1401 E 7th St.
  Charlotte. NC. USA 28204. Tel: 0172-704-375.

UK
- "Myalgic Encephalomyelitis Association"
  PO Box 8
  Stanford Le Hope. SS17 8EX. Tel: Stanford Le Hope 642 466.

Nupro (supplies a wide range of capsulated herbs, including Entrogar and Entrodophilus/Biodophilus).

Australia
- Ross Gardiner
  PO Box 559
  Manly. NSW 2095. Tel: (02) 977 0701.

USA
- Health Products International
  10 Mountain Springs Parkway
  Springville. UTAH. USA. 84663. Tel: 801-489-3635.

*Brauer Biotherapies (supplies the homeopathic Candida nosode).

Australia
- Para Rd
  Tanunda. 5352. Tel: (085) 63 2932.

USA
- Standard Homeopathic Co.
  210 West 131st St.
  Los Angeles. CA. USA 90061. Tel: 213-321-4284.
- H.R.I. Dolisos.
  6125 West Tropicana Ave.
  Las Vegas. NEVADA. USA 89103. Tel: 702-871-7153.

UK
- Ainsworths Homeopathic Pharmacy
  38 New Cavendish St.
  London. W1M 7LH. Tel: (01) 935 5330.

Alternative 'coffees' without malt*
- Health Beverage (Nature's Own)

APPENDIX

- Dendelio (Lima)
- Instant Caffeine-free Beverage (Vital)
- Old Vienna (Ralmafe)
- Rich Roast Blend (Healtheries)
- Nature's Best (Askbridge)
- Nature's Cuppa
  (For overseas readers, simply check that the alternative 'coffee' contains no malt or sugar in any form, especially lactose.)

C-Herb Tea* can be obtained from the author

- Sydney Healing Centre
  236 Darling St.
  Balmain. NSW 2041. Tel: (02) 810 6100.
  AUSTRALIA

*Candida Awareness Group

- PO Box 567
  Spit Junction. NSW 2088. Tel: (02) 819 6252.

- **USA**
  HealthComm Inc.
  3215 56th St. NW,
  Gig Harbor,
  Washington. 98335. Tel. 206-851-3943.

  U.K.
- Candida Albicans Advice Group
  P.O. Box 89,
  East Grinstead.
  West Sussex RH19 1YY

*Vai Soy (a completely malt-free soy milk and hence better than Bonsoy for people with Candida. Ask at your health food store about local brands of malt- and sugar-free soy milks)
- Vai
  29 Phillips St.
  Alexandria. NSW 2015. Tel: (02) 699 8062
  AUSTRALIA

*HYPOTHYROIDISM – THE UNSUSPECTED ILLNESS
by BRODA BARNES MD
Available from:

USA
- Cancer Book House
  Cancer Control Society
  2043 N. Berendo
  Los Angeles. CA. USA 90027. Tel: 213-663-7801

*Live Blood Analysis (blood test for Candida)

  Australia
- Australian Holistic Biologics
  2/235 Macquarie St.
  Sydney. NSW 2000. (02) 221 5488.

  USA
- Dr Bradford
  American Holistic Biologics
  1180 Walnut Ave.
  Chula Vista. San Diego. CA. USA Tel: 619-429-8200.

* Nature's Own "Hydrochloric Acid — Plus" (a supplement supplying extra hydrochloric acid for digestion)

Each tablet contains:
Betaine Hydrochloride   400mg
Glutamic Acid Hydrochloride   200mg
Pepsin   100mg

*Hiltons International (supplies vitamins by post, including product no. 127)

- Hilton House
  3 Romsey St.
  Waitara. NSW 2077. Tel: (02) 487 1155.
  Hilton's product no. 127 contains:

APPENDIX

ANTI-OXIDANTS
L Cysteine	50mg
DL Methionine	15mg
Arizona Garlic	20mg
Zinc Gluconate (Zn. 1.3mg)	10mg
Ascorbic Acid (Vit. C)	200mg
Retinol (Vit. A 10,000iu)	1.5mg
d-alpha Tocopheryl Succinate (Vit. E)	50iu
Haemoporphyrin	0.2mg

ENZYMES
Betaine Hcl	40mg
Pepsin	25mg
Pancreatin	40mg

VITAMINS
Thiamine Hcl (B_1)	25mg
Riboflavine (Vit. B_2)	10mg
Pyridoxine Hcl (Vit. B_6)	10mg
Nicotinamide	25mg
Nicotinic acid	5mg
Pantothenic acid (Vit. B_5)	10mg
Cyanocobalamin (Vit. B_{12})	25mcg
P.A.B.A.	10mg
Inositol	15mg
Choline Bitartrate	15mg
Biotin	15mcg
Folic acid	100mcg
Cholecalciferol (Vit. D_3)	200iu

MINERALS
Di Calcium Phosphate	150mg
Magnesium oxide	60mg
Ferous Fumerate	5mg
Copper Sulphate	50mcg
Potassium Chloride	15mg
Chromium Chelated (Chromium 5mcg)	50mcg
Molybdenum Oxide	100mcg
Kelp (Iodine 20mcg)	10mg

Cobalt Chloride   50mcg
Manganese Chelated (Mn 20mcg)   200mcg

HERBS
Korean Ginseng   25mg
Gotu Cola   25mg

AMINO ACIDS
L Glutamine   25mg
DL Phenylalanine   25mg

SUPPLEMENTS
Citrus Bioflavonoids   20mg
   (It contains no starch, sugar, yeast, artificial colour,
   flavour or preservative.)

BIBLIOGRAPHY

Airola, Paavo, *Hypoglycaemia — a better approach*, Health Plus Publishers, Phoenix, Arizona 1977

Barnes, Broda. *Hypothyroidism — the unsuspected illness*, Harper & Row Publishers, New York 1976

Brostoff, J. & Challacombe, S., *Food Allergy and Intolerance*, Ch. 49, Faunders Publishers. Independent Square, W. Philadelphia 1987

Budd, Martin, *Low Blood Sugar (hypoglycaemia); the 20th Century Epidemic?*, Thorsons Publishers, Wellingborough, Northamptonshire 1981

Chaitow, L., *Candida Albicans, Could Yeast be your Problem?* Thorsons Publishers, Wellingborough, New York 1985

Crook, W., *The Yeast Connection*. Professional Books, P.O. Box 3494, Jackson, Tennessee 1983

Parks-Trowbridge, J. & Walker, M., *The Yeast Syndrome*, Bantam Books, New York 1986

Gawain, S., *Creative Visualization*, Bantam Books, U.S.A. 1978

Truss, O., *The Missing Diagnosis*, published by the "Missing Diagnosis, Inc.," P.O. Box 26508, Birmingham, Alabama, 35226 1983.

Turner, R. & Simonsen, E., *Candida Can Be Beaten!*, Odium Books, P.O. Box 191 Corio. Vic. 3214, Aust. 1985

Turner, R. & Simonsen, E., *Yeast-free and Healthy*, Viking O'Neil, Penguin Books, Aust. 1987

Wunderlich, R. & Kalita, D., *Candida albicans. How to fight an exploding epidemic of yeast-related diseases*, Keats Publishing Inc., New Canaan, Connecticut 1984

WEEK 1

	SATURDAY	SUNDAY	MONDAY	TUESDAY	WEDNESDAY	THURSDAY	FRIDAY
BREAKFAST	Chicken drumsticks Steamed vegetables C-Herb Tea	Lamb's fry & onions/tomato/ sprouts Loaf/wholemeal scones C-Herb Tea	Buckwheat & rolled oats porridge Mixed nuts C-Herb Tea	Scrambled eggs Loaf toast C-Herb tea	Muesli-porridge Loaf toast C-Herb Tea	Soup Loaf toast C-Herb Tea	Fried egg Rice cakes C-Herb Tea
Memory Jogger		Soak lentils.	Defrost fish for casserole.	Defrost mince for shepherd's pie/ meatballs.		Defrost mince for chicken loaf.	
LUNCH	Tuna Salad Loaf C-Herb Tea	Soup/stew Loaf Sprouts C-Herb Tea	Quiche Salad C-Herb Tea	Mixed nuts/seeds Salad Wholemeal scones C-Herb tea	Meatballs Salad C-Herb tea	Sandwiches Salad C-Herb Tea	Kebabs Salad Loaf/scones C-Herb Tea
Memory Jogger						Defrost chicken fillets/veal cubes.	
DINNER	Roast lamb & vegetables Broccoli or salad C-Herb Tea	Dahl pancake roll Vegetables or salad C-Herb Tea	Fish casserole Noodles Vegetables C-Herb Tea	Shepherd's pie Vegetables C-Herb Tea	Omelette Silverbeet Damper C-Herb Tea	Chicken loaf Rice & sauce Pumpkin C-Herb Tea	Stuffed capsicum Salad C-Herb Tea
Memory Jogger	Remove frozen stew/soup for Sun. lunch.	Make quiche. Soak buckwheat.		Make meatballs Wed. lunch.	Defrost soup Thur. b'fast.	Prepare kebabs.	Defrost lamb chops.

WEEK 2

	SATURDAY	SUNDAY	MONDAY	TUESDAY	WEDNESDAY	THURSDAY	FRIDAY
BREAKFAST	Grilled chops/ tomato/ sprouts Buckwheat/corn pikelets C-Herb Tea	Fish Loaf/scones C-Herb Tea	Scrambled eggs & tomato Rice cakes C-Herb Tea	Pancakes C-Herb Tea	Buckwheat & rolled oats porridge Boiled egg C-Herb Tea	Mixed nuts & seeds Scones Sprouts C-Herb Tea	Chicken fillet Loaf toast Sprouts C-Herb Tea
Memory Jogger		Soak lentils or defrost mince.		Soak lentils. Defrost mixed grill.	Soak lentils.	Defrost fish.	Defrost veal.
LUNCH	Stuffed capsicum Salad C-Herb Tea	Cold chicken Salad Scones C-Herb Tea	Moussaka Scones/ loaf toast Salad C-Herb Tea	Sandwiches Salad C-Herb Tea	Savoury lentils & rice Salad C-Herb Tea	Ratatouille Salad Biscuits C-Herb Tea	Boiled eggs Salad Rice cakes C-Herb Tea
DINNER	Baked chicken Vegetables C-Herb Tea	Moussaka Vegetables C-Herb Tea	Fish cakes Salad/vegetables Damper C-Herb Tea	Mixed grill Stir fried vegetables Brown rice & millet C-Herb Tea	Ratatouille Brown rice C-Herb Tea	Fish Vegetables Kouskous C-Herb Tea	Veal casserole Brown rice Vegetables C-Herb Tea
Memory Jogger	Keep spare chicken. Defrost fish.	Left-overs for Mon. lunch.		Soak buckwheat. Prepare Wed. lunch.		Defrost chicken fillet.	Defrost chicken drumsticks.